DATE DUE

Ide‎ ‎**rom**

Identifying and Recovering from Psychological Trauma

A Psychiatrist's Guide for Victims of Childhood Abuse, Spousal Battery and Political Terrorism

by

Brian Trappler, M.D.

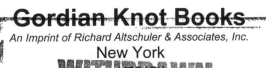

Gordian Knot Books
An Imprint of Richard Altschuler & Associates, Inc.
New York

Identifying and Recovering from Psychological Trauma: A Psychiatrist's Guide for Victims of Childhood Abuse, Spousal Battery, and Political Terrorism. Copyright© 2009 by Brian Trappler. For information contact the publisher, Richard Altschuler & Associates, Inc., at 100 West 57th Street, New York, NY 10019, RAltschuler@rcn.com or (212) 397-7233.

www.BrianTrappler.net

Library of Congress Control Number: 2009921102
CIP data for this book are available from the Library of Congress

ISBN: 978-1-884092-76-3
Gordian Knot Books is an imprint of
Richard Altschuler & Associates, Inc.

Disclaimer: This book presents the observations and treatment approaches of a board certified psychiatrist with extensive professional experience and the credentials described on the back cover of the book. The information herein is neither intended to offer precise medical advice to any given individual regarding any specific case nor to serve as a substitute for the personal advice of a licensed psychiatrist, psychologist, or other professional healthcare provider.

Cover Design and Layout: Josh Garfield

Printed in the United States of America

Dedication

This book is dedicated to:

Danny Haran and his two daughters, Einat and Yael Haran
Eldad Regev
Ehud Goldwasser
Gavriel Holtzberg
Rivkah Holtzberg

The Haran family was murdered in a terrorist attack on the Mediterranean village of Nahariya by Samir Kuntar in 1979.

Eldad Regev and Ehud Goldwasser were kidnapped by Hezbollah in a 2006 cross-border incursion from Lebanon.

After two years of negotiations, Kuntar was released by the Israeli Government in the infamous July 16, 2008 "prisoner exchange" sham. In return, Israel received the remains of Eldad Regev and Ehud Goldwasser, which required DNA identification.

Rabbi Holtzberg and his wife were murdered in the Mumbai attacks perpetrated by Islamic terrorists on the Chabad Synagogue in November 2008.

The author believes that Kuntar functioned as a consultant for the Pakistani Central Intelligence Service (CIS) during the Mumbai attacks, explaining the almost identical methodology used so effectively in the Nahariya attacks.

Although there have been hundreds of Pakistani attacks in India, the Mumbai attack was the first to target a Jewish Center and was characteristic of the sadistic and wanton cruelty that carries the trademark of Hezbollah.

Following the Nahariya attack, *Newsweek* described Kuntar's murders as "so sickening that they should give pause even to Israel's enemies." (Kuntar had forced the four-year-old Einat Haran to witness her father being shot and then drowned, before having her head crushed with rocks.)

In November 2008, Syrian President Bashar Assad awarded Kuntar the country's highest medal of honor.

Contents

Chapter 1

IDENTIFYING THE SYMPTOMS OF PSYCHOLOGICAL TRAUMA

What Is Psychological Trauma?

A *trauma* is any injury a person suffers, whether the cause is physical or emotional. *Psychological trauma* results when a person experiences a traumatic event, such as being physically beaten, verbally abused, or exposed to a terrorist attack or other horrifying event. Psychological trauma can, therefore, be thought of as an experience that overwhelms a person's capacity to protect his or her psychological integrity. Severe psychological trauma first became recognized after World War I when soldiers surviving gruesome battle scenes presented to mental health professionals with symptoms of dread, amnesia, and emotional withdrawal. Many of them were unable to return to battle.

While reading this book and thinking about "psychological trauma" and "traumatic events," it is important for you keep in mind the distinction between stress that results from threat to life and bodily integrity, on the one hand, and stress that results from less dramatic incidents, on the other hand. In other words, all traumatic events do not lead to severe psychological trauma at all times in all people. When the trauma is severe, however, it may cause you, or any person, to have longstanding distress and functional impairment.

Healthy adults with resilient coping mechanisms have innate capacities that help them to weather stress. Studies of humans, as well as on animals, indicate that after individuals experience most traumatic events, they have a brief "stress reaction" that consists of subjective symptoms, such as flashbacks, anxiety, and insomnia. These symptoms are also often accompanied by an increase in stress-mediated brain transmitters and adrenal hormones. Healthy individuals, however, also fortunately have a "stress-reversal brake-system" that restores their physiology to its normal resting state once the trauma has subsided.

As the above indicates, a "psychological trauma" is not only limited to your "mind" or "psyche" but, in fact, involves your bodily functioning and emotions. For this reason, a "psychological trauma" is best thought of as a *psychobiological* reaction to a traumatic event. On the bodily level during an extreme threat your sensory nervous system, central nervous system (composed of the brain and spinal cord), and peripheral nervous system (composed of your somatic and autonomic nervous systems) are all activated.

Although we have internal mechanisms that help us to regulate stress reactions, we also require external resources, in many instances, to help us prevent and be rescued from physical battery, sexual abuse, or other external attacks. A traumatic breach that overwhelms healthy coping-mechanisms, and disrupts normal mental, neurological, and endocrine functions, is often the result of excessive force and inadequate rescue mechanisms, either internal or external.

In this book, you will learn about all the resources you need to help you recover from psychological trauma, even if it is severe, that has resulted from childhood abuse, spousal battery, or political terrorism, among other sources of trauma. These three groups of

victims, who are the focus of this book, may share only some issues common to victims of traumas emanating from natural disasters or war combat. There *is* something unique, however, about a
trauma committed by individuals or groups against helpless civilians. Making a distinction, therefore, between interpersonal abuse
and trauma related to direct combat or events beyond our control,
such as earthquakes, makes sense heuristically, i.e., as a method
for assessing and solving problems.

Before you can seek effective external sources of help or develop internal resources to cope with and alleviate the worst symptoms of abuse or exposure to horrifying events, you need to be able
to identify the symptoms of psychological trauma. What are they
in general? Are there specific or unique symptoms commonly
found among victims of childhood abuse, spousal battery, and political terrorism? The answers to these questions are discussed in
this chapter.

Following them, in Chapter 2, I guide you through the many
types of resources you can use to recover from psychological
trauma, including behavioral therapies, "talk therapy," medication,
and meditation; in Chapter 3, I discuss seminal caretaker issues
that affect trauma symptoms and treatment in childhood; in Chapter 4, I discuss key factors that affect trauma symptoms and their
treatment in spousal relationships; in Chapter 5, I discuss political
issues that affect trauma symptoms and their treatment; and in
Chapter 6, I explain what happens to your brain during PTSD.

General Symptoms: An Overview

In this section, I will help you identify the general symptoms of psychological trauma, and the conditions that give rise to them, in as down to earth a way as possible. This is essential because all individuals suffering from psychological trauma need a language to describe what occurs in both their inner and outer worlds, as a result of their trauma, in order to understand it and seek effective treatment. While some victims of abuse seek help or treatment, many do not, for a variety of reasons. They may be unaware that they were (and sometimes continue to be) emotionally or physically mistreated, exploited, or even abused. Others simply reject help: As part of their defensive shield, they keep their personal horror stories safely guarded. Many victims resume their normal daily functions once they have recovered from the initial shock of trauma. Despite their recovery, however, at an operational level their life-quality often remains compromised.

The first challenge for victims of psychological trauma, therefore, is to identify one's unique symptoms of trauma. General symptoms are discussed first in this chapter, followed by discussions of specific symptoms associated with childhood abuse, spousal battery, and political terrorism. The second challenge is to match the trauma-generated symptoms with general diagnostic categories (discussed at the end of this chapter), since they form the basis for selecting effective treatment options, which are discussed in Chapter 2.

During the 1980s, psychiatrists began to turn their attention to an increasingly visible phenomenon: Individuals in various types of abused and traumatized groups, such as married women and victims of political terrorism, were presenting with many different kinds of problems. Mental health professionals felt a need to categorize their trauma-generated symptoms and develop appropriate treatments.

Thus far their work is best described as ongoing rather than as "completed" or definitive, since the psychological effects of severe trauma are vast, and professionals do not universally agree about the full range of effects generated by psychological trauma. Since the odds are so great that any person will experience psychological trauma during his or her lifetime, experts have had to set a *threshold of who qualifies* as a "trauma victim." In fact there are several trauma-generated conditions, each quite unique, and I will guide you through them in this chapter.

Some symptoms of trauma are quite striking while others are difficult to identify. The matter is made more complex by fundamental differences in trauma symptoms that exist among different types of groups, such as military combatants, victims of political terrorism, survivors of natural disasters, and victims of childhood abuse and spousal battery who have suffered prolonged, interpersonal abuse in everyday, domestic situations. In addition, newly identified victims of chronic deprivation and abuse continue to teach us—with their personal horror stories—just how evasive, yet disabling these symptoms may be.

Despite mental health professionals' lack of universal agreement about how to identify and categorize symptoms related to psychological trauma, they are now forging a growing, general consensus about how best to explain trauma symptoms and place them into reliable diagnostic categories. This approach, based on research findings from many independent investigators, allows therapists from various backgrounds and schools of thought to successfully apply their central theories of causality and treatment to assist victims suffering from psychological trauma.

In this chapter, I discuss virtually all the symptoms that occur in the lives of trauma sufferers, as well as the unique, modal symptoms experienced by victims of childhood abuse, spousal battery, and political terrorism.

In general, trauma symptoms extend from transient distress to serious derailment of normal ego-functions, depending on the severity of the individual's abuse, be it mainly psychological, emotional, physical, or sexual; the individual's age or stage of the life cycle; and factors such as temperament and personal faith, which require more research to fully understand.

Victims of severe trauma may present themselves for help to doctors or therapists with a variety of complaints. They may even be unaware that their authentic psychological world still lies buried somewhere in the past, frozen at the trauma scene. For these victims, life—somehow, unknowingly—has ceased to unfold in a spontaneous joyful way. Despite recent breakthroughs in our understanding of biological markers in trauma, there is no simple test to confirm the diagnosis of psychological trauma. Clinicians will identify trauma-related symptoms and then judge whether the victim's level of distress or functional impairments meet the requirements for a particular diagnosis.

Identifying the General Symptoms of Psychological Trauma

Dissociation

The most extreme, immediate response to trauma is *dissociation*, or a condition in which a person's awareness and ability to engage psychologically in the present is temporarily lost. When some people are presented with a threat that leads to intense fear or horror, for example, their consciousness (or awareness) "escapes" them. Since this type of trauma is emotional, not physical, they don't actually "lose" consciousness. Rather, it is as if their brains are telling them, "I can't deal with this" and, magically, their psyche "parks" itself somewhere in "metaspace," or "limbo." This displacement of the traumatized individual's integrated awareness can range greatly in terms of both severity and duration.

The most common and benign indicator of dissociation is *amnesia*, which exists when the trauma survivor has difficulty recollecting the details of what happened during the trauma. Sometimes the person with amnesia will retain only memory fragments of the trauma incident, which are insufficient to synthesize into a coherent trauma narrative.

A more serious form of dissociation is the *"fugue state,"* where the victim experiences total disorientation following a traumatic event. Well-documented cases abound in the trauma literature of survivors of catastrophic events found wandering around confused and unable to identify themselves. This form of severe dissociation, with temporary identity loss, is at the extreme end of the "dissociative spectrum" of disorders.

Among those with dissociative disorders of various types and degrees are survivors of prolonged interpersonal trauma, such as childhood or spousal abuse. These victims may emotionally "tune out" in such a way that others identify them as merely "distracted," "detached," or "emotionally absent."

This phenomenon represents a form of "structural dissociation," according to Pierre Janet, a pioneer in the area of hypnosis research. Janet's explanation for this phenomenon is that the trauma has split the personality into separate compartments, which function independently. One most often finds this in victims of chronic abuse, where victims compartmentalize their "emotional self" from their "false self." According to Janet, this "defense" allows the individual to partially engage the world in an operational way (the false self) while defensively detaching the emotional self. While this form of repression may be adaptive in some circumstances, "structural dissociation" represents a permanent structural split in the personality of these damaged trauma survivors.

The most serious manifestation of structural dissociation was formerly termed "Multiple Personality Disorder" and then renamed as "Dissociative Identity Disorder." As vividly depicted in the film *The Three Faces of Eve*, the essential feature of this disorder is the presence of two or more distinct identities that recurrently take control of the individual. Each personality has a distinct name, personal history, and identity. While this condition is now considered quite rare, there are some clearly documented cases. They all objectively confirm that these individuals had past histories involving physical or sexual abuse.

In summary:

1. Dissociation is an automatic response to an overwhelming feeling.

2. Dissociation is an experience where a person becomes unconsciously removed from the present environment.

3. Dissociation is usually triggered by fear and allows the person to escape unbearable emotional pain.

4. To an external observer, individuals "shut down" as they lose touch with their sense of being anchored in the present while becoming absorbed by the trauma recollection.

5. Structural dissociation can have a compartmentalizing effect on the structure of the personality. This, too, is at an unconscious level, meaning the individual does not identify it as a problem.

Fear

Fear—one of the most powerful, primary negative emotions—is a common symptom of psychological trauma. When people are gripped by fear, they feel "afraid" or "anxious" or "apprehensive" about a possible or probable situation or event. Even a single, catastrophic event, such as being beaten up or sexually abused, can sometimes overwhelm the "fear circuitry" of the brain.

According to Edna B. Foa—a renowned, international authority on the psychopathology and treatment of anxiety and post-traumatic stress disorder (PTSD)—people who have been chronically traumatized experience a "blurring" of their traditional boundaries between safety and danger. Their world becomes dominated by a "fear paradigm," in which life is reduced to a constant state of fear and dread. For such victims, once a trauma violates their safety assumptions, they subsequently experience the world as being constantly unpredictable and uncontrollable.

This situation is made worse because traumatizing experiences have a tendency to "generalize" onto other aspects of life, and thus sensitize individuals to a widening array of new "threat cues." Situations previously considered safe become danger signals. This increases the likelihood that traumatized individuals will constantly be scanning the world around them to identify threats to their safety and well-being. Their *sympathetic nervous system* (SNS) is constantly on the alert. In this state of activated threat arousal, there is a greater likelihood of interpreting ambiguous information as dangerous, by which they become constantly re-traumatized.

Research on "fear conditioning" shows that individuals subjected to horrific events react with both heightened emotions and avoidant behaviors when subsequently confronted by similar events. Once individuals become fear-conditioned, a vast array of "triggers" becomes capable of exacerbating trauma recollections and autonomic overarousal. "Stimulus generalization" is, therefore, integral to the so-called "fear cascade." Exposure to these trauma triggers subsequently unleashes the full cascade of traumatic symptoms.

While living in a state of apprehension and perceived threat may be adaptive for most trauma sufferers, for example, by helping victims of battery avoid potentially dangerous situations, this is not the case for victims of PTSD. They continue to function in a "survival mode" even when the threat has been removed. These individuals show a narrowed attention focus, constantly scanning the world for threatening information.

At a biological level, fear arousal in the brain results in the production of toxic neurotransmitters, which impair the functioning of the Hippocampus. This is the brain structure responsible for memory synthesis and recall. It is a memory-structure that contains information about fear-relevant stimuli, interpretations of the fear stimulus, and adaptive response choices. It is the key structure that allows the victim to process traumatic memories in a constructive way. This structure is only able to maintain its resilience if the trauma is of manageable intensity and duration. Failing this, continued arousal and stimulation by stress-produced neurotoxins shuts down this integrative function, preventing the consolidation of the trauma into a coherent narrative. From a cognitive psychology perspective, the neurobiology of the role of the Hippocampus in fear and trauma is further discussed in Chapter 6.

Suffice it at this point to mention that an activated state of threat arousal that overwhelms the victim's ability to "self-soothe," and remain "anchored" and "mindful," will prevent the victim from accessing and reprocessing traumatic material.

Avoidance

It is easy to understand why any person, or other intelligent organism, would flee from a direct threat or even "threat association"—for the sake of self-preservation. Avoidance behaviors have the effect of terminating the unpleasant feeling of fear or dread—and they are learned. Instrumental learning, in particular, is a fundamental concept for understanding avoidance behaviors. With this type of learning, we come to act in a certain way that is rewarding. In other words, we learn to respond in a way that is *instrumental* for producing a change in the environment that we find beneficial or rewarding. This mechanism explains why we avoid internal painful memories and external trauma triggers.

When stressful *overarousal* persists, however, so does the avoidance response. This situation sets up a pathological dichotomy: On the one hand, if a person's inhibitory control is not strong enough, then "flashbacks" and "arousal" emerge. On the other hand, if inhibitory mechanisms over-assert themselves, then avoidance symptoms dominate.

People tend to avoid not only when they perceive external threats, but also when they experience painful affects and memories, which are internal. Paralleling this external/internal source of stimuli, the avoidance mechanism may have both unwanted external and internal consequences. Externally, it deprives the victim of the joy of "creative engagement" in the world. Internally, it narrows the victim's full range of emotional experiences. For this reason, victims of any form of chronic trauma may appear to others as emotionally distant, restricted, or absent.

For patients with PTSD, psychiatric professionals now believe that to extinguish fear and overarousal, the patients must fully recount their trauma story, i.e., they must communicate all components of their "trauma narrative" to the therapist. When the "avoidance defense" is active, it helps people ward off frightening memory fragments and painful affects but, at the same time, it allows these fragments and painful affects to simmer in the unconscious. The avoidance defense thus stifles memory and plays a role in denying patients access to all aspects of their trauma story. The result is that this process contributes to the chronic nature of PTSD.

Flashbacks

A flashback is a sudden, vivid recollection of any past trauma experience. While people usually "see" flashbacks—that is, experience them visually—they can also "hear" them, experience them as emotions, such as fear or anger, or even experience them as physical sensations, such as pain.

Flashbacks can occur spontaneously, when survivors are reexposed either to internal trauma recollections or external trauma triggers. They can also be induced both by hearing about the traumatic event (that is, by exposure to trauma narratives) and seeing visual imagery associated with the traumatic event—including computer-generated virtual reality scenes.

Flashbacks also may take the form of nightmares. I have had Holocaust survivors as patients, for example, who had become sleep-phobic because they experienced predictable visitations of images, sounds, or smells of the crematoriums in the concentration camps. Such experiences torment these survivors, since flashbacks are experienced as if they were happening in the present.

When one has a flashback, one doesn't black out; but one does take temporary leave of the present and travel to the past trauma, reliving it, even believing that the traumatic event is happening all over again. For this symptom to occur, the traumatized individual exhibits a deficiency both in "self-soothing" and "anchoring" functions. If the victim also has a significant reservoir of "split-off" (or unmetabolized) trauma material, this easily resurfaces. Both of these aspects need attention in the recovery process, and are discussed in Chapter 2.

Negative Interpersonal Schemas

As we grow up from infancy, each of us forms mental pictures— "templates" or "models"—of relationships with others, which I refer to as an "interpersonal schemas." They are based primarily on our early relationships with parents or other caretakers, and influence the dynamics of our future relationships with others.

Victims of interpersonal abuse usually have *negative* interpersonal schemas that carry over into their lives as they grow older, and tend to be re-enacted. Eventually those individuals, abused during childhood, tend to relive the traumatic events in their adult lives.

According to the therapeutic school known as "Cognitive Therapy," abuse schemas subsequently sabotage all interpersonal relationships. The victim's schemas will later translate into miserable or dysfunctional relationships, and such individuals live in a world where to be "attached" means to be "abused."

The basic elements of the abuse-generated schema are the following:

- Children have a normal instinct to seek attachment and comfort—even from bad caregivers
- Models learned within the context of traumatic relationships become programmed into the brain, and are called "interpersonal schemas"
- These schemas guide subsequent expectations and behaviors in future interpersonal situations
- Childhood abuse distorts and disrupts the formation of healthy schemas
- Abused or neglected children carry these distorted schemas into adulthood
- These schemas might continue to influence your experiences and feelings about relationships and events throughout your life
- They can inadvertently result in patterns of repeated negative relationships
- You may be easily exploited, or feel helpless to stand up against predators
- Such schemas have to be reshaped in recovery

Identifying and changing unhealthy relationship patterns are central to the reversal and disruption of these abusive patterns. Such patterns have to be replaced by one's capacity to feel safe, confident, and empowered in all relationships. The achievement of this goal frees the individual from the compulsion to "act out" past traumas in the present.

What Is Meant By "Self-Agency"? Do You Have Issues With Power Failure or Submission?

Throughout life, if most of your relationships were abusive, then your ability to relate to others would be within a narrow range of expected outcomes. All new relationships would likely follow a narrow focus of appeasement and obedience. You may become confined in relationships to giving up all of your rights and self-dignity in order to remain *attached*.

Your abuse-generated survival tactics may, in fact, be maladaptive in the larger world. You may not feel entitled to self-regard, respect, and affection. You may continue to be abused by authority figures, and lack the skills to identify or free yourself from this negative attachment to others. If you are a woman, for example, you may find men to be sexually exploitative or degrading, yet you cannot be assertive or disrupt your participation in such relationships. The notion of escape overwhelms you with fear. You cannot express your personal rights for fear of retaliation. You cannot perceive an alternative way to move beyond this narrow script.

In general, you may feel that your relationships lack spontaneity and fluidity. You cannot articulate your goals or make life choices until you transcend your recurring trauma narrative. You have been robbed of the opportunity to enjoy the full landscape of social freedom.

Confronting these maladaptive self-schemas and reclaiming self-agency is a vital component in the recovery of Complex Trauma, and will be discussed in Chapter 2 on treatment options.

Emotional Dysregulation

Emotional *regulation* refers to people's capacity to tolerate all kinds of emotional states while feeling comfortable in their own skin and positively engaged in life. Victims of severe or prolonged psychological trauma, however, are more likely to feel they are living in a world dominated by internal emotional turbulence or *dysregulation.*

For example, if you were abused as a child, you are not only more likely to constantly feel negative, but trivial events are more likely to upset you. You are also less able to neutralize these feelings or "self-soothe." If you lack the capacity to neutralize unpleasant feelings, they are prone to erupt in the form of angry outbursts. Alternatively, you may escape overwhelming distress by numbing your emotions with illicit drugs.

Effective emotional regulation contributes to more fulfilling relationships, work-effectiveness, and parenting. Strategies for regulating emotions are learned throughout development, but are primarily embedded in early development by our parents or other caretakers. Healthy maturation allows one to face negative emotions in relationships by holding onto good internalized objects, such as parents, which have a soothing and containing effect. When this capacity is lacking because of early neglect or abuse, victims are more likely to continuously re-experience and re-enact their early abuses without any emotional safety-buffers.

Trauma-Related Syndromes

From the above discussion, you can now identify the individual *symptoms* of psychological trauma, which can potentially afflict any given individual who has been the victim of abuse, battery, assault, terrorism, or other traumatic event. It is also important that you understood how these individual symptoms sometimes cluster together or develop into different kinds of syndromes. A *syndrome* can be defined simply *as a group of symptoms and diseases that together are characteristic of a specific condition.* In this section, I will describe what psychiatrists call "trauma-related syndromes," in increasing order of seriousness and complexity.

Despite the diversity of symptoms produced by all types of psychological trauma, most symptoms will conform to and can be described by the following categories:

1. Stress-related Symptoms
2. Acute Stress Disorder
3. Post-Traumatic Stress Disorder (PTSD)
4. Complex Stress Disorder, or DESNOS (Disorder of Extreme Stress Not Otherwise Specified

Stress-Related Symptoms

Most survivors of a shocking event will develop some *stress-related symptoms* such as feeling frightened, jumpy, and easily startled. The survivor's sleep may be fretful, concentration becomes impaired, and assumptions about personal safety are replaced by uncertainty. Although these symptoms are common and may be highly stressful, they are usually benign.

An acute trauma might occur in all of the victims who are the focus of this book. In child abuse, the violation may range from excessively harsh acts of "punishment" to any sort of sexual molestation. In domestic abuse, the weaker partner usually becomes the "victim" of physical or sexual assault. In political trauma—which we usually associate with acts of violence against any ethnic group—the violation can range from individual hate-crimes to large-scale attacks on societies.

Following an attack on an individual or community, the majority of survivors (plus witnesses, perhaps) are prone to the following reactions:

- Biologically, the sympathetic nervous system becomes temporarily over-activated
- The individual remains in a heightened state of vigilance. This may last from a few hours to days
- The victim worries about the personal safety and whereabouts of significant others

To counter this stress reaction, emotionally healthy individuals summon various coping mechanisms and engage in certain behaviors to reduce their stress. The following is a list of some adaptive behaviors generated by the stress-reaction:

- Communication with others about what they have experienced
- Establishing contact with significant others using cell-phones
- Trying to get an idea of the "big picture" via TV, radio, and Internet
- Seeking confirmation that safety and order have been re-established

- Seeking emotional soothing via bonding and communicating with others, even strangers

Later, the healthy survivor will try to "put it all together." This process is what trauma therapists call "creating a *trauma narrative*."

Other factors that will lead to containment of the stress response include the following:

- When parents assure young children "everything is all right," because children need such reassurance (children also closely monitor their parents' level of alarm)
- When one has been sheltered or immunized against previous trauma
- When the duration of trauma-exposure is relatively brief
- When social infrastructures are maintained (these include safe access to food, shelter, and medical assistance)
- When timely and efficient rescue interventions are provided
- When there is effective governmental leadership
- When there are strong social supports

Once these conditions are met, most individuals will rebound psychologically and continue with their lives relatively unscarred. This is what occurs in cases when an assault is contained by a combination of robust internal and external resources.

Acute Stress Disorder

Now let's focus on traumas that result when all lines of defense are penetrated. This overwhelming situation may result from seemingly simple factors, such as the magnitude or frequency of the trauma. In such circumstances, or where the victim has remained vulnerable to recurrent boundary violations by the predator, personal or collective chaos ensues, stress mechanisms become overwhelmed, and the surviving victim is prone to a multitude of problems.

Acute stress disorder is a serious response to a shocking violation or near-death experience. It begins within hours or days after a traumatic event, and the victim suffers a combination of *dissociation* as well as the full-blown spectrum of post-traumatic stress symptoms, which is discussed shortly below.

A minority of survivors experience a dramatic disruption of their state of awareness following an overwhelming trauma, called *dissociation*. In the *dissociative* state (discussed above), survivors experience a disruption in their ability to integrate the flow of consciousness and remain focused on what is occurring. They are also unable to re-establish emotional containment. This situation usually results in a "shutting down" effect. Psychiatric researchers suspect that the biological underpinning of this phenomenon is a temporary loss of synthetic brain function that predominantly involves the Hippocampus and Pre-Frontal Lobes (see Chapter 6 for definitions of the brain components involved in psychological trauma).

If the victims also have flashback symptoms, marked anxiety, or hypervigilance and attempt to run away from ("avoid") anything (even thoughts) that remind them of the experience, then psychiatrists calls this syndrome *Acute Stress Disorder*. These symptoms usually occur when people are directly exposed to and threatened by a *horrifying* event.

Sometimes victims of Acute Stress Disorder experience dissociation so severe that they present to mental health professionals in a *trance-like state.* I witnessed this first-hand in the Emergency Room at SUNY Downstate, Brooklyn, which was designated a Disaster Treatment Center within hours after the 9/11 terrorist attacks on the World Trade Center Twin Towers. As the Attending Psychiatrist on call, I evaluated several patients rescued from the Twin Tower buildings, as follows:

One young woman had been walking down the stairwell when she heard a tremendous explosion. She quickened her pace until she smelled fumes and heard screaming. At that point she opened the door and stood on a small platform (all that remained of that floor). Immediately, a burning tire came hurtling down, missing her by inches. As she gazed up, she saw above her the remnants of offices, disconnected from their main landing, like suspended islands. Injured and burning survivors, assured of their pending doom, could be seen screaming in pain and terror.

The woman paused before realizing that their fate was sealed, and then continued down about another 40 floors until reaching the exit. She remained in the chaos at "Ground Zero" for a short time, and then followed a crowd of people walking across the Brooklyn Bridge. Several hours later she arrived home in a "dazed state." Her mother brought her to the Emergency Room the following morning. She had paced the floor of her apartment the entire night without sleeping.

On evaluation, what one observed was a young woman who was staring blankly in front of her. She was quietly moaning and sobbing. She was still totally immersed in the trauma scene as if it were occurring that moment. Not only did she not answer questions, she didn't even notice my presence in the room. From time to time she would reach or call out to the victims still visible in front of her. On several occasions she raised her hands to shield herself against falling debris.

This evaluation depicts the most extreme form of dissociative reaction, where the victim was so fixated to the scene of the trauma that the "present moment" in time did not exist for her. These symptoms are obviously more serious than the "stress-related symptoms" of being afraid and worried, which I discussed earlier in this section.

If the symptoms recounted above for Acute Stress Disorder persist beyond four weeks, then professional intervention is usually required, since the individual would now have evolved into the more persistent condition of *post-traumatic stress disorder*. (See Chapter 6 for details of the biological disruptions that occur in PTSD.)

Post-Traumatic Stress Disorder (PTSD)

What is PTSD? I will attempt to first illustrate this diagnosis with the following trauma vignette, taken from my article in the *American Journal of Psychiatry,* "Post-traumatic Stress in the Survivors of the Brooklyn Bridge Shooting."

In 1994 there were several acts of terrorism targeting Jewish civilian populations around the globe. This included the bombing of the Jewish Community Center in Buenos Aires, a terrorist attack on a cafeteria in Jerusalem, and the suicide bombing of a bus in downtown Tel Aviv. Lubavitcher Hasidim living in Crown Heights, Brooklyn, represented a vulnerable target for a terrorist attack because of the Lubavitcher Rebbe's outspoken position on Middle-East politics.

On March 1, 1994, the Lubavitcher Rebbe, considered by many Orthodox Jews as being the spiritual leader of world Jewry, underwent ambulatory surgery in Manhattan. Returning to Crown Heights, his ambulette was accompanied by an informal convoy of cars and vans. As a security, the convoy split into two columns. Instead of returning to Brooklyn via the Brooklyn Bridge, the Rebbe's vehicle was deliberately detoured via the Brooklyn Battery Tunnel.

As the rest of the convoy entered the ramp to the Brooklyn Bridge, a white van carrying 15 yeshiva students was ambushed by a Muslim gunman. One student was killed instantly and another critically injured with a bullet wound to the head. Approximately 30 bullets were fired into the van. In the ensuing chaos, one student tried to control the profuse bleeding from a head wound to the student next to him. The gunman, who drove his car alongside the van for the length of the bridge, continued firing at close range using two semi-automatic pistols. Two additional students were wounded in the ensuing chase, one receiving a serious bullet wound to the abdomen.

I evaluated and began debriefing 11 of the survivors within 24 hours of the attack.

Together, with Dr. Steven Friedman, the students underwent clinical and psychometric examinations prior to and at the completion of 10 weeks of trauma group therapy. Survivors of the shooting were compared to an age-matched sample of classmates of the van group.

Of the 11 students studied in the trauma group after four weeks, four of them met criteria for PTSD in the *Diagnostic & Sta-*

tistical Manual-IV (or DSM-IV). Four other students showed significant elevations of stress including anxiety and depression, while three survivors did not meet criteria for a DSM-IV diagnosis.

The DSM-IV is the psychiatric manual used in America to diagnose emotional disorders, while the Europeans use the "ICD-10" (*International Classification of Diseases–10*) to classify all emotional disorders. For the DSM-IV, it suffices that a victim has been "confronted" with a traumatic event (meaning even as a witness) that evoked an emotional reaction characterized by intense fear, helplessness, and horror. This definition would, therefore, include even rescue workers. The IDC-10 is stricter in that it requires *direct exposure* to an event of an exceptionally threatening nature that "would evoke distress in almost anyone."

For the students discussed above who were suffering from PTSD, the most distressing symptoms were visual flashbacks, dissociative symptoms and hyper-arousal. Avoidance symptoms were the most persistent, with most of the terror victims showing extreme reluctance to travel the Brooklyn Bridge. Several needed continued exposure therapy after the completion of the 10 formal group therapy sessions.

The above-mentioned attack on a group of students is one of many trauma occurrences where the psychometric testing showed stress elevations in *all* of the victims of the shooting. But PTSD developed in approximately one-third of the students. In addition, one-third suffered from other stress-related symptoms, and one-third failed to meet any DSM-IV diagnosis.

While the victims' PTSD symptoms persisted for 8 to 10 months, they were no longer causing emotional or social difficulties after two years. Since other studies have shown persistence of symptoms after two years, improvement in this group might have been due to early intervention and the emotional support of a close-knit community.

Despite the "popularity" in the media of PTSD—which is depicted in many movies and TV shows and discussed in many books and magazine articles—it is somewhat misleading to believe that PTSD is the exclusive, prototypic response to serious psychological trauma. In fact, there are many different reactions to trauma—a full array of reactions to various types of trauma exposure—which are described throughout the course of this chapter.

While PTSD constitutes only one of several possible reactions to abuse or trauma, it remains the traditional cornerstone of the serious psychological effects of trauma.

In addition to experiencing three groups of symptoms—intrusive thoughts, avoidance, and hyper-arousal symptoms—there is a consensus among experts regarding the required severity of trauma, or the "trauma-threshold." This threshold is necessary to distinguish PTSD victims from the rest of the population who undergo the stress of daily living. Both the IDC-10 and DSM-IV classification systems require the trauma victim to have endured a terrifying or potentially life-threatening event.

The following domains of symptoms, then, need to occur to satisfy the requirement for the diagnosis of PTSD:

1. Intrusive symptoms, such as flashbacks, nightmares, recurrent thoughts or images about the trauma

2. Avoidance symptoms, whereby the individual steers his or her life away from trauma-reminders: staying isolated from anything associated with trauma dominates this defensive mode of behaving. Included in the "avoidance" domain of symptoms are even

those defensive efforts made to ward off thoughts or feelings about the trauma.

3. Hyper-arousal symptoms, whereby the individual's neuro-biological state is shifted to one of generalized hypervigilance. The victim now experiences the world within a "paradigm of fear."

If traumatized individuals continue to experience persistent distress due to the three above-mentioned domains, they meet the criteria for PTSD as defined by the DSM-IV manual of psychiatry. A partial review of some pertinent neurobiological aspects of PTSD can be found in Chapter 6.

Complex Trauma

This section identifies the silent suffering of victims of repeated or prolonged trauma, no matter the cause. There was a time when psychiatrists and other mental health professionals attempted to fit all trauma-related symptoms into the single category of PTSD. Several years after PTSD was adopted by the American Psychiatric Association, in the DSM–III, as *the* stress disorder, several land-mark publications revealed that this diagnosis captured only a lim-ited scope of post-traumatic symptoms.

Various studies of traumatized children, for example, reported patterns of unmotivated aggression and lack of impulse control, attentional and dissociative symptoms, and difficulties negotiating interpersonal relationships. Other investigators studied victims who had survived rape or incest during childhood. Their findings, too, illustrated problems not captured in PTSD. Instead, these vic-tims appeared to have a compromised sense of safety, self-worth, and capacity to regulate emotions or "self-soothe."

People who have been in any type of prolonged abuse situa-tion, including hostages, children, and spouses, may continue to feel and behave as if they were still victims—because the sense of danger they felt when they were in the abusive situation never passed from their consciousness, awareness, or memory. Throughout their lives, they describe themselves as feeling "emotionally dead inside," and other people see them as being detached. The explanation for this symptom is their failure to develop or maintain adequate *self-caretaking* functions required by any individual to feel emotionally whole, which are strengthened each day by positively engaging the world.

From a "Self-Psychology" perspective, these victims have been robbed of their "good self-objects" and, as a result, cannot "self-soothe." From a "Cognitive Psychology" perspective, these victims are unable to remain "anchored" and "mindful." Experts in the field of trauma have made extensive efforts to capture the full list of individuals' "self-functions" that are disrupted when they have been exposed to extended abuse and political terror. In Chapter 3, I describe the role of normal and required parenting, which I also frequently refer to as "caretaking."

The other symptoms and disorders mentioned above surprisingly appear to have received little attention until 1992, when Judith Herman discussed them in her monumental book, *Trauma and Recovery*, which described the "expert consensus" of studies of survivors of child abuse. Almost 20 years after all psychological effects of trauma had been squeezed into the label of PTSD, there emerged a new term for this syndrome: "Complex Trauma."

Judith Herman described the following symptoms in patients with prolonged histories of high-magnitude, inter-personal trauma: (a) disturbances in perception of self and others, (b) a propensity to repetitive patterns of trauma re-enactment, (c) an inability to regulate mood, and (d) even the adoption by victims of the belief systems of their tormentors.

Other investigators in the field of *prolonged interpersonal trauma* described these victims as experiencing one or more of the following three symptoms: a loss of coherent sense of self, an inability to engage in stable or trusting relationships, and an inability to free themselves from the abuse dynamic. While some victims became abusers themselves, others appeared to become compulsively attracted to predators. By so doing, they continued a "repetition-compulsion" of their childhood abuse into their adult relationships.

Prior to identifying the disorder of *Complex Trauma,* patients presenting with disturbances of attention (including dissociation), affect-regulation, and interpersonal relationships (including serious character pathology) had been labeled with "diagnoses not recognized as being trauma-generated." In fact, experts had long-expressed their concern of limiting the construct of trauma to "PTSD." The most notable downside of the narrow PTSD paradigm was the exclusion of a diagnostic label for trauma-victims presenting with some of these other important trauma-generated symptoms. These victims would not reap the benefits of emerging therapeutic modalities crucial for trauma-recovery. Indeed, patients presenting with trauma symptoms outside of the narrow PTSD construct were not even asked about trauma or abuse! In a recent review article in the *Journal of Traumatic Stress* about instruments clinicians use to screen adults for PTSD, Chris Brewin reported that none of the 13 identified instruments currently in use were found to include items that rate Complex Trauma.

The emergence of Complex Trauma into the field of trauma psychology opened the floodgates to a wide spectrum of new symptoms that affect personality structure, mood regulation, belief systems, and interpersonal behavior. Considering that these trauma-generated symptoms govern essential and enduring psychological functions, they appeared to be even more far-reaching than PTSD in their complexity and implications for treatment.

As a result of this increasingly obvious omission, researchers established a DSM-IV "field trial" (or study in the natural environment rather than a laboratory). It explored the notion that prolonged trauma, particularly at an early age, may have significant effects on psychological functioning above and beyond PTSD. The DSM-IV PTSD field trial included a review of the literature on trauma in children, female victims of domestic violence, and concentration camp survivors, and it identified 27 items belonging to seven of the domains listed below. These items were later used to compile the "Structured Interview for Disorders of Extreme Stress," or "SIDES."

According to a report in the *Journal of Traumatic Stress* by David Pelcovitz et al. (who also conducted the field trial), all three groups of subjects who had experienced prolonged or high-magnitude exposure to interpersonal trauma showed significant elevation on the SIDES scale. These trauma victims were labeled as suffering from *Disorder of Extreme Stress Not Otherwise Specified* (*DESNOS*) by the DSM-IV task force. Over time, this terminology became synonymous with "Complex Trauma." It appeared that a new diagnostic entity had been successfully fashioned. As a diagnostic syndrome, it highlighted problems not captured in PTSD, particularly targeting victims of rape and incest, battered women, and victims of political terror or genocide. This new diagnosis includes the following seven categories proposed by Judith Herman:

1. Alterations in regulation of affect and impulses
2. Alterations in attention or consciousness
3. Symptoms of a somatic nature
4. Alterations in self-perception
5. Alterations in relations with others
6. Alterations in perception of the perpetrator
7. Alterations in systems of meaning

This new diagnostic entity now provides a legitimate format for victims of continuous trauma who present with a spectrum of functional impairments not incorporated by PTSD. Complex Trauma addresses the following eight self-functions that may have been damaged by the traumatic experience:

1. The capacity to feel secure and emotionally comfortable in relationships

2. The capacity to feel empowered in relationships with others (via empathic engagement)

3. The skills required for self-awareness

4. The skills required for affect-regulation and self-soothing

5. The personal sense of boundaries

6. The ability to preserve world beliefs and a sense of meaning

7. The ability to stay "anchored" and "mindful" during stress (as opposed to dissociating)

8. The ability to tolerate a full range of emotions without being overwhelmed or shutting down

A Personal Note on Complex Trauma and DSM-IV

Rather than being separated into a new diagnostic entity expressing the core areas of damage in the chronically traumatized population, the condition known to experts in the field as "Complex Trauma" unfortunately became relegated in the DSM-IV to a sub-category of PTSD. This inclusion of "Complex Trauma" as a sub-diagnosis or complication of PTSD would prove to be problematic, because many victims of chronic trauma and abuse do not have PTSD.

Julian Ford, from the National Center for PTSD, writing in the *Journal of Clinical & Consulting Psychology,* distinguishes the cardinal symptoms of chronically abused adults, especially when the abuse had occurred at a young age, from the symptoms of PTSD. In his study of 84 patients admitted to a specialized inpatient PTSD Residential Rehabilitation Program, Ford found that PTSD and DESNOS represented two distinct clinical syndromes. Ford supports the conventional knowledge that exposure to combat alone results in fear, avoidance, numbing, and hyperarousal, which are the cardinal symptoms of PTSD. However, symptoms of Complex Trauma were not found in pure samples of combat survivors, but were only associated when the trauma occurred early or there was atrocity participation.

While conceding that the two trauma groups do show an overlap of symptoms, battered children and spouses, incest survivors, POWs, and survivors of genocide, torture, terrorism, kidnapping, and war atrocities usually have symptoms better characterized by Complex Trauma or "DESNOS." These symptoms include extreme affect and impulse lability, self-fragmentation, pathological dissociation, existential confusion, and interpersonal conflict due to compromised core object-relations.

While victims of child abuse are more vulnerable to developing signs of Complex Trauma or (DESNOS) in the face of ongoing abuse, severely mistreated adult populations, such as POWs and survivors of genocide or continuous threat, are also at risk for developing symptoms of Complex Trauma. In fact, many trauma survivors who do not meet PTSD diagnostic criteria display substantial DESNOS symptoms. Ford also did not find PTSD to "fundamentally impair psychological development or core object-relational capacities."

I am, therefore, in agreement with those who argue that "Complex Trauma" become a completely independent diagnostic entity in the Trauma section of DSM-V.

As you can see from this chapter, symptoms of trauma range from brief stress reactions to complex changes in personality function that are deeply embedded and have long-lasting effects on a person's life.

In the remainder of this chapter, I discuss symptoms of psychological trauma most commonly found among victims of childhood abuse, spousal battery, and political terrorism.

Victims of Childhood Abuse: Identifying Symptoms of Psychological Trauma

Some aspects of trauma symptoms are unique to *young* victims. Childhood is a time when the individual is most vulnerable to victimization. The internal personal resources with which adults protect themselves are limited in children, because of their still underdeveloped cognitive, affective, and physical resources. As a result, children may not be able to recognize, avoid, or protect themselves from predators.

Trauma in childhood may range from punitive parenting habits to severe cases of battery. Abused children often lack the resources of adults, either to find a place of safety to recover or to muster social support networks. On the contrary, children have little choice about where they live or on whom they depend for their safety or survival. Their home is the traditional source of safety but *this very place* can—and too often does—become the setting of their injury.

To escape, an abused child has to run the risk of telling an *outsider* about his or her parent's or other caretaker's abuse. This act carries the frightening implication of loss of home, caretaker, and the danger of retaliation for the betrayal.

Furthermore, gaining access to appropriate rescue agencies and institutions that will effectively protect the child is almost impossible for children to do alone.

The implications of childhood abuse by a caretaker-turned-perpetrator is quite staggering. The safe attachment of a child to its parent is fundamental. It is the cornerstone and foundation for the child's development. From this relationship will evolve a sense of agency, self-definition, autonomy, self-regulation, and templates for relationships otherwise known as "cognitive schemas." A distorted early attachment will function as *the* template for the child's future sense of self and the world around him or her, as discussed above in this chapter.

When a child's traditional source of safety becomes the very source of danger, the damage is most likely to cause long-term changes in any of the above-mentioned personality functions described in the section under "Complex Trauma." In contrast to adults, however, abused children often confound the effects of abuse by their ambivalent love-hate feelings toward their caretakers.

Abused children also carry certain additional burdens:

- They may become trapped in a maze of conflicted feelings toward their caretakers
- They may lie or conceal their injuries to protect their caretakers
- They may believe that what is happening to them is normal
- They may not know how to access external resources for rescue

A child's healthy attachment to the parent or other caretaker is also critical for an adequate sense of security to explore and engage the world. Abusive parenting robs the child of the assets necessary for gaining a sense of mastery and autonomy.

According to experts in Complex Trauma, such as Daniel Siegel and Mary Hartzell, authors of *Parenting from Inside Out*, when children develop secure attachments with caretakers they feel inwardly confident. As a result, they are empowered as adults and function as a safe haven to others. This not only stabilizes self-functions, but also is required in subsequent relationships with others, in particular with one's own children.

As emphasized by Jennifer Freyd in *Betrayal Trauma*, a lesson needs to be learned from each tragic case of caretaking failure. Any form of child abuse is an essential betrayal by the caretaker that prevents the child from developing these essential assets. The following is a partial list of the enduring consequences of child-hood abuse:

- The loss of sense of security and personal safety
- The loss of the ability to trust
- The loss of the ability to engage in intimate relationships
- A sense of shame and guilt (instead of a sense of well-being)
- An impaired capacity to love oneself
- An impaired capacity to soothe oneself
- A diminished capacity for true empathy towards others
- A distorted belief system
- A distorted perception of self and others
- A deficient capacity for focus and recall
- An impaired ability to modulate anger
- A poor sense of effectiveness and personal agency
- Chronic somatic complaints

The consequences of betrayal trauma may be seen in the following anecdote drawn from my own practice:

I was requested many years ago by the Office of Mental health to oversee the visitation of a 14-year-old boy by his father. The boy had been placed in custodial care of his grandparents by the office of "Special Services for Children" (S.C.C.).

This situation began when a schizophrenic mother of five children battered her first son into a coma. The son miraculously survived, and was allowed to return to his parents with weekly visits by a social worker. The father, in my opinion, was mildly retarded with a schizoid personality. The extended family's priority was to keep the authorities out of their business. Whatever family problems did occur was covered over, so that after one or two years the family was discharged from S.C.C.

The mother, however, remained poorly controlled psychiatrically. She had frequent outbursts of unexplained rage, which she would take out on her husband or children. Her husband spent as much time away from his wife as possible, to escape her psychotic rage.

No professionals remained involved to monitor the impact of the mother's schizophrenia *on the household* once the case was closed by Protective Services. There was a treating psychiatrist whom she would visit periodically to renew her medications. The psychiatrist was not provided with collateral information needed to grasp the "big picture."

One day her husband arrived home from work to discover that his younger son had been bludgeoned to death.

His wife received a prison sentence of about seven years. The husband was put on probation and allowed to visit his children, who were placed under the grandparents' supervision.

In actuality, the father's "crime" was that he lacked the intrinsic skills to be a caretaker. He was not an angry, punitive or violent man. But he was an "enabler" and passively colluded with the ongoing abuse that he witnessed.

In fact, in his limited way, he loved his children. But he showed poor judgment in leaving the children unsupervised and was, therefore, guilty of negligence.

In my opinion, the truly guilty parties, after the first, near-fatal assault, were the agency caseworkers and supervisors. *They* failed to protect the household from a persistent threat. This negligence, combined with the silent complicity of the father and grandparents is, in fact, what led to the death of the child. This case illustrates how internal and external resources can fail when an abusive family is sheltered by a tightly-knit, closed community.

Investigators in the field of trauma are focusing their attention on how to recognize survivors of habitual abuse. Their symptoms may be either physical, emotional, or a combination of both.

Physical symptoms include the following:

- Children who are undernourished
- Children who are inadequately dressed
- Children showing signs of physical assault
- Children persistently late for class
- Uninvolved parents

Emotional symptoms include the following:

- Children who have difficulty concentrating in class
- Children who appear distracted
- Children who are emotionally withdrawn or detached
- Children who do not interact playfully
- Children making vague excuses to protect their parents

While young survivors' trauma symptoms may escape immediate detection, they will later surface in a variety of different ways as more discernable symptoms of what we now recognize as Complex Trauma.

Childhood abuse should also be ruled out when the patients are adolescents presenting to mental health professionals with disorders such as Substance Abuse, Eating Disorders, Somatoform Disorders, and Dissociative Disorders (which the DSM-IV refers to as "Axis I Disorders").

Victims of relentless abuse may show signs of severe *personality disorders*, such as "borderline" or "antisocial" personalities. These trauma symptoms are embedded within the victim's personality, and are classified in the DSM-IV as "Axis II Disorders." On closer scrutiny, many of these individuals appear to have unsuccessfully repressed their histories of childhood abuse.

In contrast to the above-described victims, children who are victims of a solitary event—such as rape—present with symptoms of Acute Stress Disorder or PTSD, and are usually *very distressed* about their symptoms for which they seek help. Indeed, following a single episode of physical or sexual violence, a child, like an adult, may present with symptoms of severe distress, including confusion or dissociation. This may also lead to classic PTSD.

These more evasive, long term effects on core personality development, now classified under the category Complex Trauma, are currently believed to be the most frequent and worrisome outcome of childhood abuse, rape, or any form of prolonged, life-threatening trauma. Such victims of prolonged, interpersonal trauma often present to mental health professionals with the kind of symptoms and relationship disturbances that seem to belie any causal relationship to their abuse histories and, therefore, escape detection. However, they cause immense suffering, since the abuse may thwart personal development and contribute to interpersonal failures in multiple areas of functioning.

Victims of Spousal Battery: Identifying Symptoms of Psychological Trauma

For victims of spousal abuse, like victims of childhood abuse, their psychological trauma begins and continues within the traditionally safe environment of the home. The kinds of abuse they experience and suffer from range from constant verbal criticism to restrictions on friendships to outright physical and sexual assaults.

Predators—including spouses and others in intimate relationships—like to isolate their victims. Within spousal relationships, there are "benign abusers" who dominate their relationships through a pattern of control and criticism. This type of abuse is not gender-specific, i.e., wives or girlfriends can control or abuse their husbands or boyfriends in several ways. This dynamic is well illustrated in the movie "Misery" starring Cathy Bates, where, it turns out, the predator is a female. Indeed, I have seen a man of giant stature not only emotionally abused but also "emasculated." Some wives tyrannically rule their men and control them like children. In reality, gender becomes secondary when the victim-to-be chooses (subconsciously) to live out this abused role, based on a deep-rooted psychological "victim-predator schema." Unless this trauma schema is identified and uprooted, the victim will continue to find or construct a spouse who perpetuates the trauma dynamic.

Although spousal abuse is "gender neutral," generally speaking, when most people think of spousal abuse they conjure up the classic image of an aggressive male pummeling his fragile wife or girlfriend into submission. In the remainder of this section I will focus on the more violent forms of abuse and use the male pronoun "he" for simplicity as well as to capture the fact that most violent abusers are, in fact, male.

Spousal abuse usually occurs in a predictable cycle that culminates in actual violence. The cascade usually begins with a "trigger." For example, the victim speaks in a tone or behaves in a way that makes her husband feel she's defied her subservient role. The triggers provoke anger in the abuser, which leads him to retaliate against his victim. The retaliatory response may range from a tantrum, to that of a threat, a shove, or a full assault. The spectrum of responses may vary, depending on the trigger, the extent of perceived insubordination, and the level of anger and impulse-control of the perpetrator.

This cycle usually terminates with some form of token remorse and reconciliation toward the wife. His "make-up" behavior combined with her fear of punishment or abandonment, however, contributes to her sense of ambiguity, indecision, and *inaction*—as we saw in the case of Nicole Simpson, who was battered and probably killed by her husband, O. J. Simpson, according to the civil jury that found him liable for her death.

In ways difficult for outsiders to comprehend, the wife-victim of spousal abuse often remains ensnared in the relationship with her husband-predator—since she is gripped by a pervasive sense that "there is no way out."

Most abusive husbands have learned to hide what they are doing to their spouses, by mastering the skill of living a "double life." The "good" predator, in fact, is often psychopathic in his ability to disarm neighbors, employers, peers and even family, by appearing as the "model citizen." But in the private world of his home, he is intimidating and dangerous. Usually it is only the victims who see their spouse's dark side expressed in its "full glory."

The typical abuser uses several of the following tactics to impose the trauma dynamic on his victims:

- He attempts to isolate his spouse from others. This tactic disconnects the victim from *rescuing resources*
- He may track his wife's telephone calls or listen in on conversations to assure his victim's loyalty and obedience
- He establishes a relationship in which there is no notion of "power-sharing"
- He conveys an unspoken understanding of "who is the boss" and the painful consequence that will ensue should his wife not "play by the rules"

Behind the public facade, the victim's playfulness is replaced by a constricted countenance. Embroiled in this dynamic, joy and optimism are replaced by caution; social engagement is replaced by shyness and inhibition. When concerned friends and family members attempt to explore the problem, the victims offer a predictable array of rationalizations and platitudes to conceal their imprisonment at all costs.

This system of unspoken rules often characterizes all forms of interpersonal abuse, be it at the individual or collective level. Abusive spousal relationships often proceed unchecked for three major reasons. First, the victim may be too frightened, confused or ambivalent to act decisively, escape or get help. Second, legal bureaucracies are too slow and cumbersome to deter a crime of passion. Third, government agencies prefer to have domestic problems solved within a "community" by the community.

I have seen "cover-ups" in all communities, unfortunately, sometimes for reasons that are held to be in the best interest of the "community" rather than the individual. All of us, in fact, are aware of cases of spousal battery, along with cases of child molestation, covered up by religious sects to protect the "community's image." Only in the most egregious cases do governmental agencies engage these issues.

Victims of Political Terrorism: Identifying Symptoms of Psychological Trauma

While acts of childhood and spousal abuse that result in trauma are committed against individuals, acts of terrorism have the ability to violate the safety and well-being of entire societies, replacing order with insecurity, fear, and, ultimately chaos. The U.S. State Department (2008) defines terrorism as "premeditated and politically motivated violence perpetrated against non-combatant targets," i.e., innocent civilians.

The most tragic instances of terrorism involve acts of genocide or ethnic "cleansing," where entire populations of civilians are annihilated or "purged," such as during the Holocaust or more recently in Rwanda.

Modern terrorism disseminates fear and dread across communities and even entire nations, often by usurping the vast network of mass media and transmitting trauma imagery to every corner of the world. The continuing threats, goals, and capabilities of modern terrorists and their state sponsors have profound mental health implications for tens of millions of people everywhere.

Politicians, educators, therapists, and concerned citizens are encouraged, therefore, to understand the psychological and political ramifications of terrorism in as much depth as possible. In this section, I will discuss the full array of symptoms suffered by individuals who have been exposed to terrorist attacks, based on both my own experiences treating victims of terrorism and findings from published studies on populations recently exposed to terrorist attacks.

In both witnesses and survivors of a terrorist attack, we can see what happens to normal civilians confronted with something shocking, catastrophic, and totally unanticipated. While survivors of these events may suffer a wide array of benign symptoms, such as worry and apprehension, a minority develops signs of serious psychological trauma.

An example of a terrorist attack that resulted in high-intensity, short-term trauma for tens of millions of people, especially those living in New York City, occurred just after the Twin Tower terrorist attacks on September 11, 2001. A few days after the attacks, 44 percent of a nationally representative sample of adults reported high levels of stress in at least one of five substantial stress categories, while 90 percent reported at least some levels of stres.These findings of traumatic stress symptoms stretched *across the entire nation.* However, the closer people lived to Lower Manhattan, the more likely they were to suffer from *significant* stress symptoms. Those who spent many hours each day watching the event on television also developed stress reactions, even though they personally experienced no direct threat to their lives. This phenomenon is referred to as the "vicarious stress syndrome." While a majority of residents in New York City experienced substantial stress levels in the weeks following the 9/11 terrorist attacks, the New York Academy of Medicine reported a prevalence rate for full PTSD of only 7.5 percent after 5 to 8 weeks and only 0.6 percent after 6 months.

At the epicenter of a terrorist attack, 90 percent of surviving victims may exhibit some adverse psychological reaction in the hours and days following the critical event. While the frequency of psychological distress dissipates as one moves in time or distance from the epicenter, a small but significant percentage of previously healthy individuals continue to bear significant distress. Such findings were reported in demographic studies conducted with local and national populations exposed to trauma imagery. Following the 9/11 terrorist attacks, for example, national surveys of stress reactions by Schuster et al. and Schlenger et al. identified substantial symptoms of stress in Americans across the country. Similar findings were reported from studies conducted after the Madrid and London train and bus bombings, which occurred soon after the 9/11 attacks on the Twin Towers.

These findings contrast, however, with the levels of stress-related symptoms found in a study by G. James Rubin and associates on the London populace after attacks there by Islamic terrorists on July 7, 2005. The results showed that 31 percent of the population reported substantial stress levels in the weeks following the attacks. Of particular interest in this study was that Londoners with previous exposure to Irish Republican Army (IRA) terrorism appeared more immune to distress. This suggests that gaining mastery over previous traumatic events may immunize one against future exposure to such events.

The frequency of "stress-related symptoms" in London was, however, much less than that observed after the 9/11 New York terrorist attacks, where emotional distress was experienced not only throughout the United States but also around the world, especially in political allies of America, such as Britain, Israel, and Italy.

One can understand the severity of distress following the 9/11 attacks. Several of the icons symbolizing America's prowess as the world's "superpower" were demolished within about one hour. The event changed the world as we knew it. For the first time ever, Islamic Jihad demonstrated that the United States was *vulnerable*.

Follow-up studies of trauma survivors demonstrate that most victims "habituate" over time, i.e., they develop a certain tolerance or diminution of trauma-induced symptoms. A small but significant percentage of them, however, remain in a state of hyper-vigilance, and are distressed by the visitations of traumatic recollections or "flashbacks." These victims also often engage in a variety of avoidance behaviors, in an unconscious attempt to shield themselves against further trauma triggers, which in itself can become quite disabling.

Moreover, previously traumatized populations are prone to a *recurrence* of symptoms when exposed to a new trauma, even after many years. This has been confirmed by several studies of re-traumatized populations. According to a study conducted by David Kinzie, for example, Bosnian and Somali refugees seeking refuge in the USA from their war-torn countries of origin suffered a much higher frequency of PTSD than native New Yorkers following the 9/11 attacks; and Israeli Holocaust survivors suffered much greater stress after the Scud missile attacks in the Gulf War than the rest of the elderly Israeli population. These and similar findings indicate that factors such as the severity and duration of trauma and the victim's age, support system, and previous exposure to trauma, among other factors, determine the severity and outcome of symptoms.

As previously mentioned, the most extreme, immediate response to trauma is *dissociation*, where the individual's awareness and ability to engage psychologically in the present is temporarily lost. A minority of trauma survivors experiences this dramatic disruption of their state of awareness; this *dissociative* state reflects a shift in the survivor's integrated flow of consciousness and synthetic brain function. For those survivors who are more vulnerable to the effects of trauma, or those exposed to a stress of unusually high intensity or duration, the world freezes at the trauma scene and subsequently ceases to unfold in a spontaneous, cohesive way. If an individual exhibits dissociation together with flashback symptoms, marked anxiety or vigilance, and attempts to run away from ("avoid") anything (even thoughts) that reminds him of the traumatic experience, then psychiatrists diagnose the individual as having Acute Stress Disorder.

These symptoms are obviously more serious than the frequent occurrence found in the majority of single-trauma survivors, referred to as "stress related symptoms," where survivors complain of being afraid and worried.

If the symptoms that compose "acute stress disorder" persist beyond four weeks, then the trauma effect has probably evolved into that of *post-traumatic stress disorder* (PTSD).

When a society is exposed to enduring or repeated attacks, then the population is likely to continue to feel vulnerable, which results in a state of chronic vigilance. That is the purpose of terrorism: to make a population feel helpless or defenseless against an invisible predator and, thus, highly anxious or fearful. Once such a fear paradigm has been established, entire communities are likely to be afflicted with the symptoms of Complex Trauma, which Arieh Shalev has termed the "Continuous Threat Paradigm."

Once a pattern of continuous threat or intimidation is established (whether in the form of child or spousal abuse or political terrorism), it disrupts individuals' psychological functions and social behaviors in a far more sinister way than any single event. People living under prolonged conditions of threat show deficiencies in their sense of "personal agency." They are fearful something horrible might happen again in the future and thus more avoidant in their behaviors. (See the discussion of Complex Trauma above for a more detailed discussion of these symptoms.)

A good example of this syndrome comes from several studies on trauma among Jews and Arabs in Israel, conducted by the Israeli Trauma Center for Victims of Terror and War, since the controversial Camp David and Oslo "Peace" Accords. In one study, Avi Bleich reported that after 44 months of Intifada, *half* of the Israeli population felt their own lives and those of their friends and families were in danger.

Terrorists, in fact, purposely use the "continuous threat paradigm" as an integral part of their methodology. To achieve this end, many of the recent terrorist attacks have included the following components;

- Dramatic visual dissemination of barbaric acts, such as the attacks on public transport systems
- Attacks on national icons, such as the Twin Towers and Pentagon
- Kidnappings of aide-workers, clergy, and journalists
- Public beheadings of high-profile civilians, such as the journalist Daniel Pearl and the American contractor Nick Berg, in Iraq
- Assassinations of pro-democracy political figures, such as Harik Hurari and Benazar Bhutto

- Car bombings in highly populated locations, such as shopping markets, cafes and recreational centers

The cumulative effect of this terrorist methodology is to make people feel afraid, insecure, and generally unsafe. At the same time, the terrorists use the news media to announce their presence and agenda to a worldwide audience. Having established a methodology of fear conditioning, populations may be targeted by the terrorists to be intentionally humiliated or even forced to parade their shame. An integral part of this Jihadist strategy is also to coerce the victims to publicly accept and promote their kidnappers' propaganda. This was demonstrated when Iran captured a British naval boat in international waters, then mockingly paraded the English sailors before an international audience. The supposed "caretaker" in this situation (the British Government) colluded in this public national humiliation before the world audience.

Subjugating and humiliating individual victims and even entire nations gratifies a collective, sadistic need, which is intrinsic to the methodology of radical Islam. The moral weakness, confusion, and ambivalence of current Western civilization has created a climate ideal for the fermentation of political tyranny and the spread of terrorism. This information is quite disturbing, since it leaves entire communities vulnerable to abuse, not unlike a helpless child without a caretaker, who is left to the whims of a predator. See Chapter 5 for a detailed discussion of the emerging role of caretaker failure in political terrorism.

Chapter 2

RECOVERING FROM PSYCHOLOGICAL TRAUMA

An Overview of Resources and Methods

In this chapter, you will learn about various ways you can alleviate or fully recover from the symptoms of psychological trauma. They include natural or self-healing, self-soothing, anchoring, emotional regulation techniques, the help of a professional therapist, and medications. The various paths to recovery I discuss in this chapter apply regardless if your trauma was caused by childhood abuse, spousal battery, political terrorism, or any other factor or process. What is most important, I believe, in choosing the best path to your recovery, is understanding if your psychological trauma is a "Type I" or "Type II" Trauma (described later in this chapter). This distinction, above all else, should determine the treatment modality trauma survivors choose, and I will devote a good deal of attention to this in the pages that follow. No matter what accounts for your reduction of symptoms, however, I believe it is important for you to understand some general principles, concepts, and ideas involved in the healing process, so that you can maximally recover, remain symptom-free, and cope with "flashbacks" and "triggers" as they occur throughout your life.

Understanding General Principals, Concepts, and Ideas in Trauma Recovery

Extricating Yourself from a Traumatic Situation

In order for you to recover from psychological trauma, it is almost essential that you first extricate yourself from your traumatic situation, if at all possible. If you are a victim of spousal battery, for example, it is necessary that you remove yourself from that situation before therapy or another possible solution can effectively resolve your trauma. In some instances, however, it is not possible for trauma victims to remove themselves from a situation, such as U.S. soldiers stationed in Iraq or civilians living in the Middle East, where attacks are possible at any given time. In those instances, it is possible that some trauma victims may have a "natural" trauma recovery (which will be explained below), but for others, recovery will be difficult if not impossible.

Once survivors have been rescued from any immediate threat, then they need to feel safe and confident enough to understand what happened to them, so that they can "put the matter to rest."

An example of this is illustrated in the case of the classic, violent, jealous, physically dominant, male predator, where the victim has to establish whether the aggressor is a "Trickster" or a true psychopath. (See the discussion of Carl Jung's archetypes in *Ego and Archetypes* by Edward Edinger.) The trickster might posture, threaten, and intimidate, but he counts on his antics as the means to overpower his victim. In such a scenario, the victim, if resolved to escape, should succeed because the trickster might be putting on an impressive show via deliberate tactics of intimidation. The victim, however, is fighting for her survival. In such circumstances, the victim may be able to free herself by cleverly out-tricking her predator.

Occasionally the predator is extremely dangerous, by which I mean a psychopath, felon, or pedophile. In such circumstances, you may constantly be in mortal danger, unless you obey the rules and constantly prove your loyalty. From a psychological perspective, you can only empower yourself by plotting your escape very carefully and with total resolve.

Strategies to accomplish this goal would include:

- Establish a safe and totally private sanctuary
- Change your cell phone number
- Have only your most trusted person know your number
- Don't choose someone your predator would expect
- Communicate only with crucial contacts via a third person
- Find an aggressive attorney who understands your predicament
- Make all contacts with the predator via your attorney or a law enforcement agency
- Do not have contact with your predator directly, in person, by email, or on the phone

The Importance of the Caretaker Function

If you, an innocent citizen, have been victimized as a result of your caretaker's malicious behavior or negligence, then, of course, your normal assumptions about trust and safety have been challenged. The experiences people suffer that fall under the category of abuse range from early emotional deprivation to constant verbal criticisms to physical assaults to sexual violations.

Sometimes caretakers collude passively in the abuse, rather than actively, yet in so doing they allow or even enable the abuse to continue. An example of this is the case I described earlier of a schizophrenic patient whose husband—as well as the Child Welfare caseworker and psychiatrist—allowed her to be with her children without supervision, which resulted in negative consequences for the child victim.

This principal has political and social significance. A caretaker's primary responsibility is to protect the welfare of the individuals or communities under their trust. This moral responsibly applies to the parents of a child, the mutual caretaking between spousal partners, or, at a collective level, a government towards its citizens.

Mental health professionals involved in trauma healing have to, before anything else, begin the process of *allowing the victim to believe that the world is safe again.* The *empathic bond* established early in therapy may constitute the first building block in replacing your sense of chaos and danger with that of order and predictability. The microcosm of safety in the therapeutic relationship, however, can only be effective if it is supported on the outside by a safe, social infrastructure or *"holding environment."*

In the case of child abuse, appropriate education of "first-responders" must lead to sensitive but effective social intervention. The daughter of one of my schizophrenic patients, for example, would arrive in school inadequately dressed in the winter, which was ignored by adult authorities. She later developed anorexia, and was finally hospitalized. The mother was secretive about her husband's violent outbursts because she was terrified that the child would be removed from the home. Finally, the school principal notified the psychiatrist. The child was allowed home after she reached her critical body weight, but the after-care procedure included monthly reports by the visiting social worker to a mental hygiene court without disrupting the child's school and social environment.

In relationships characterized by a perpetrator-victim dynamic, there is sometimes no real safe haven for the victim. Such victims, having never been properly soothed, may never learn the capacity to self-soothe. For this reason, trauma therapists need to be kind, supportive, and empathic. For the healing process to succeed, victims need to have an emotional sense of being "held," or comforted, by others. This makes it easier for victim-patients to share their stories in the comfort of "someone who is on their side." Gradually, patients are able to internalize this sense of safety they feel with the therapists as becoming part of themselves. This outcome empowers victims to begin to engage the world with a sense of personal efficacy.

The Trauma Narrative

Most unrecovered trauma victims remain "stuck" in the unresolved narrative of their trauma. That is, you must be able to resolve the "story" (narrative) you tell yourself about your trauma, before you can wholly or largely recover. Once you correctly process your narrative, then trauma will no longer torment you. Until that time, most trauma victims will need to devote their resources to try to ward off spontaneous painful recollections, or else they will be consumed by the painful emotions and flashbacks they elicit. In Type II Trauma victims, the unresolved trauma narrative may carry over into trauma reenactments.

The victims of Type II Trauma, when exposed to trauma triggers, are more likely to experience symptoms belonging to the Complex Trauma syndrome. In particular, situations that remind victims of their predators will cause them to feel helpless and vulnerable, as if they were becoming victims in the present. Victims of childhood abuse, for example, are constantly re-traumatized by other males who are aggressive or authoritarian. This causes them to regress into their childhood victim roles, because of the carry-over effect of unresolved trauma. It is important to distinguish between the present threat, which is merely a trigger, and the original trauma process. The narrative will involve resolution of the original traumatizing situation. In fact, the trigger functions as a helpful probe that your therapist can utilize to assist you in uncovering your repressed trauma material.

Engaging the Present and "Dual Awareness"

As a result of this internal inferno, you may not be able to engage the *present* in an unfolding spontaneous way. In fact what is occurring in the present may have little relevance to you. Dedicating your resources to warding off trauma triggers will inhibit your ability to spontaneously engage the present.

For trauma survivors to begin liberating themselves from *reliving the past in the present* (through fear, anger, or painful recollections), it is crucial for survivors to believe that they can realistically do so safely: *There is no clear and present danger.*

If you are working with a professional therapist in the trauma recovery process, then it will be incumbent upon the therapist (or other helping agency) to regain your trust that has been lost.

In the process of trauma healing, *dual awareness* is a skill you can acquire that will enable you to revisit your trauma within a safe "holding environment," armed with a new repertoire of techniques to manage the discomfort generated by re-exposure to your trauma. This capacity to move freely in your mind between the *safe present* and *dangerous past* is generated by building *dual awareness,* to safely navigate between the safety of the present reality and the terror of past memories.

All trauma practitioners and theorists, no matter what their "school of thought" or tradition, are in agreement that this dual awareness will require you, as a survivor, to "revisit the crime-scene" of your personal trauma. In one form or another, you will have to face your past horror in order to fully engage the present with a sense of safety.

Self-Soothing

During the healing process, the ability to "self-soothe" will be helpful, through any safe means that works for you. This might include exercise, painting, meditation, yoga, martial arts, dance, or religious practice, among many other possibilities. The capacity to self-soothe is largely determined by early developmental factors, especially your parents' success in having soothed you. This process will be discussed more fully below. Rational choices for escape are greatly enhanced when a victim acquires techniques such as "anchoring" and "mindfulness." Self-soothing functions are also crucial for brain structures to perform the tasks required in synthesizing trauma narratives.

The Caretaking Function and Personal Agency

What is unique about the three groups who are the subjects of this book—victims of childhood abuse, spousal battery, and political terrorism—is that the traditional sources of comfort and security have failed them. In trauma recovery, the cornerstone of treatment is providing an environment that is physically and emotionally safe. Only when convinced by an empowered, *benevolent care-*

taker (such as a psychiatrist or trauma recovery group) can victims begin to safely re-establish their sense of *personal agency*.

The feeling of safety must encompass the survivor's social, political and religious life, where the umbrella of protection encompasses a newfound confidence of expression, in an environment free from external threat. This confidence will need to be constantly reconfirmed that it is indeed safe to engage in new patterns of thinking that allow you to assert and express your own belief-system. This is a huge change compared to when you were in a traumatic situation; for in order to maintain control over your destiny, your predator considered it of paramount importance to let you know that any attempt at autonomy would have dire consequences.

In a therapy or helping group relationship, the therapist (or group members) will give you affirmation for positive gains you have made. This process, proposed by Margaret Mahler, a leading developmental psychologist, uses concepts such as *hatching* and *rapprochement* as crucial tools people can call on for recovery. A healthy parent, for example, by allowing a child to individuate while responding supportively to any frustrations the child experiences when leaving the safe-haven of the caretaker to engage the world, will later buffer the child against external trauma.

Many traumatized individuals lack this confidence and sense of well-being required to protect themselves against the exploitations of predators. These skills now have to be learned and applied using newfound supports. Your original parent or other caretaker laid the foundation for determining your feelings of safety, self-worth, sense of agency, and ability to assert your personal rights in any relationship. You will now have to summon these resources to free yourself from the external triggers that have controlled you.

The trauma therapist will function as a catalyst to create a safe holding-environment that will mobilize rescue functions.

This concept also applies at the collective level, where protective social and governmental agencies play the parental role in protecting citizens from internal (domestic) or external (terrorist) threats.

External Helping Resources

You will also need to muster the skills to mobilize external helping resources. These include access to food, shelter, medical supplies, schools, work, and other social and community networks. In domestic and political terrorism, predators usually attempt to isolate their victims. Social and governmental caretaking agencies shoulder the burden of identifying victims and providing access to these external helping resources. This should be particularly stressed in the case of abused children, who may never have developed the skills to independently access these resources.

Type I (Acute) Trauma and Individual Therapies

Trauma experts generally agree and accept that the school of "Behavioral Therapy" has the most evidence-based data to support their treatment modality for acute ("Type I") traumas. This modality, which consists of "forcing" trauma victims to *relive* their trauma in each session, is also referred to as "exposure therapy." Trauma experts came to appreciate that the full benefit of exposure therapy is applicable to victims of single trauma events (i.e., Type I events). In this type of therapy, during each session the therapist guides you to relive your trauma via imagery or narration. Each time you confront the trauma, your distress will lessen, until most of your anxiety is extinguished. This phenomenon is also referred to as "extinction" or "habituation."

An expanded spectrum of behavior therapy referred to as "Cognitive Behavior Therapy," is discussed more fully below. This spectrum constitutes a large repertoire of *cognitive* therapies available to train you, as a victim, to employ "self-help" strategies that allow you to face trauma-triggers without being overwhelmed by excessive fright.

Not all survivors remain sufficiently calm and focused, however, to build a coherent narrative out of their trauma: When confronted with trauma reminders, many victims continue to experience exacerbation of fear and threat. Severely traumatized victims need to learn a variety of other coping strategies before they are able to withstand re-exposure to severe trauma triggers. For instance, in my research on Holocaust survivors, I discovered that many of my patients never discussed their experiences in the concentration camps, even with their spouses and children. It becomes critical, therefore, to recognize the entity known as Complex Trauma, which often is found to be resistant to traditional exposure techniques.

The Rationale for Bio-Medicinal Treatments

Recent biological advances in the understanding of trauma have also lead to a more rational approach of medical treatments. Biologically, when the emotional (limbic) brain is overly stressed, it becomes overwhelmed with neurotoxic stress hormones. As a consequence, it loses its capacity to perform the multiple complex tasks required to integrate a "trauma-narrative." It is of paramount importance, however, to switch-off the over-activated stress-response, sometimes medically, before irreversible damage occurs in the Hippocampus. Medications that are effective in treating Type I trauma are discussed shortly below. This integrated approach of biological and psychological interventions needs to be strongly emphasized. When required, medication can lower the arousal thermostat, which allows the limbic brain to benefit from these new coping strategies.

Type II (Complex) Trauma

The new approach to trauma recovery focuses on a wide range of target symptoms. The exposure of the entire range of abuse has opened the window to the study of emerging treatments in severely traumatized victims. The spectrum of symptoms and treatments for trauma has mushroomed with the recognition of the entity of Complex Trauma. Marylene Cloitre, a renowned trauma therapist, has proposed strategies to teach chronically-stressed victims new skill-sets that can *restore* the brain's resilience. Today's target symptoms involved in Type II, or Complex, trauma go beyond "conditioned fear" and include symptoms such as "alterations in relations with others" and "alterations in sense of meaning," which are prevalent in Complex Trauma victims. Using instruments such as the "Structured Interview for Disorders of Extreme Stress" (SIDES), therapists can measure these other deficits in self-functioning caused by chronic trauma.

Stockholm Syndrome. The list of Complex Trauma treatment strategies is now wide enough to even include conditions such as the well-known "Stockholm Syndrome." In this condition, the victim identifies with the predator and actually accepts the "new meaning to life" imposed by the predator. In the recent past, we have seen this phenomenon imposed on large population groups by communist and fascist dictators, and today we see it in many cults and, especially, in fanatical Islam. Accepting tyrannical ideologies as "truths" has facilitated the dissemination of the propaganda-template of the predator while nullifying the victim's sense of personal autonomy. When your predator strips you of your authentic personal sense of meaning, you lose the capacity to critically self-reflect. Once the victim has re-established his or her sense of boundary, it becomes the task of the trauma therapist to convince the victim that it is safe to have personal beliefs, even those not popularly held, without the threat of retaliation. Perceptions and meanings of self and others that have been altered by coercion should be re-examined following rescue from any hostage-type relationship. Trauma recovery (particularly Type II), therefore, requires personal scrutiny of all of the ideas and ideologies imposed on you by your previous predatorial masters.

Mindfulness and the Therapeutic Relationship

Therapeutically, you can use the strategies of "mindfulness" not only to calm yourself (anchoring) but also to restore your capacity for self-observation. The process of mindfulness ranges from *recognizing* when you're "losing it" (to fear or anger) to becoming aware of *triggers* that cause you either to have distorted perceptions or develop unwarranted trauma-generated feelings of guilt, shame, or vulnerability.

With regard to recognizing the symptoms of acute or chronic trauma, the victim and therapist need to be aware of "trauma-re-enactments," which are often displayed by abuse victims throughout their lives and even within the therapeutic relationship. Distorted perceptions, in particular, can profoundly distort the relationship between trauma victims and their therapists; for example, victims may be prone to see their therapists as the "depriving" or "abusive" parent. In radical contrast to this perception, some victims of abuse perceive their therapists as "saviors." This can become particularly burdensome to therapists. In general, the more that trauma victims lack the ability to self-soothe or regulate their emotions, the more likely they are to bring substantial interpersonal distortions into the therapeutic relationship.

This is the predominant focus in the "Psychodynamic" school of therapy, where therapists use the analysis of this "transference" (e.g., when the victim-patient sees the therapist as a "parent" or "savior") to help trauma victims gain insight into their emotions and patterns of behavior in other close relationships. Trauma therapy also borrows skills from the "Dialectic-Behavioral" school, founded by Marsha Linehan, where treatment is particularly relevant in victims of childhood abuse who develop serious distortions and trauma re-enactments. Today this approach is the cornerstone in the treatment of individuals with "borderline personalities," many of who were abused as children.

As stated or implied throughout the above overview, the healing of trauma contains many elements, which include diverse schools of treatment methodologies. In the following sections of this chapter, I will discuss the various types of therapy mentioned above in more detail, including Behavior Therapy, Cognitive Therapy, Self-Psychology, Psychodynamic Psychotherapy, Dialectic-Behavior Therapy, and Trauma Group Therapy. In addition, I will discuss the role of medication therapies in the treatment of psychological trauma, other types of "alternative" treatments, such as meditation, and social rescue functions that allow victims to begin the path to recovery from trauma.

Two Distinct Types of Trauma:
Type I and Type II

As stressed above, from a therapeutic perspective the types of trauma that you, or any trauma victims, can suffer may be divided into two distinct trauma categories that require different treatment approaches: Type I ("Acute" Trauma) and Type II ("Complex" Trauma). Each type of trauma is consistent with a certain kind of event, process, or situation that produces the expected reaction.

Type I Trauma Victims

A Type I traumatic event produces a reaction consistent with a sudden, unanticipated threat of death or injury. This trauma is sometimes referred to as a "critical incident." It can occur in victims of childhood abuse, spousal battery, or political terrorism. In childhood or spousal abuse, the critical incident may consist of a physical or sexual assault. In political terrorism, the type of event would be that of a terrorist attack. The commonest type of attack is the "suicide bombing," such as was perpetrated on 9/11 and subsequently on the transit systems in Madrid and London.

The *mildest* form of Type I symptoms belong to the category of Stress Related Symptoms. These symptoms include worry, insecurity, and poor sleep, which are reported by most individuals in the immediate aftermath of any attack or assault.

The *most severe symptoms* of Type I Trauma are found among individuals with PTSD, which is an *ongoing* disorder characterized by physiological overarousal, intrusive symptoms (such as flashbacks), and avoidant behaviors.

Treatments for these symptoms range from peer-support (in mild cases) to Behavioral Exposure Therapy. Treatment has to emphasize the need to *contain* the emotional "shock," "switch down" the excitation of the sympathetic nervous system, and restore some kind of emotional stability within several days, to prevent cell death in the Hippocampus associated with PTSD.

During the initial period of stabilization, the trauma victim may require a combination of rescue resources, empathic support, physical relaxation, or temporary use of calming agents such as minor tranquillizers (discussed in the section on "Medications"). The objective of the treatment is to reduce victims' levels of distress, arousal, and avoidance or numbing.

Type II Trauma Victims

In contrast to a Type I Trauma, a Type II Trauma refers to prolonged or repeated trauma at an interpersonal level, such as occurs with longtime victims of spousal battery or childhood abuse. A Type II Trauma does not produce the dramatic symptoms of a Type I Trauma, with its "shock" effect on the arousal system.

Rather, the presentation of symptoms to therapists is often delayed, and the symptoms *mimic* those of attention disorder, dissociation, social adjustment disorders, anger management problems, and distortions of belief-systems.

Although being hostage to a controlling or punitive parent or spouse or living under the fear of tyranny or terrorism may not cause individuals to exhibit symptoms as dramatic as those among Type I Trauma victims, the former type of victims may likely be living with and suffering from a complex set of impaired self-functions. For this reason, they may require long-term psychotherapy to address their characterological impairments, such as Cognitive Therapy or Self-Psychology. While the former will identify the specific deficiencies, the latter will concentrate on re-establishing safety and well being.

When Type II Trauma occurs early in childhood, the effects are more profound. But most victims of chronic abuse present with deficits in core personality functions (see the discussions of "Complex Trauma" and "Childhood Abuse" in Chapter 1).

Type II Trauma Victims with Symptoms of Type I Trauma

Some victims of trauma present themselves to therapists with symptoms of both Type 1 and Type II Traumas. For instance, a sexually molested child may suffer from acute symptoms of distress or even confusion (Type I symptoms), but after continued exposure to abuse ("repetition of the abuse dynamic"), the child may later develop Type II changes in core self-functions. In other words, child victims subjected to atrocities are more likely to suffer from PTSD (Type I Trauma symptoms) initially, and later show serious personality disorders (Type II Trauma symptoms).

I know about such children first-hand, through my professional practice. For example, I supervised a psychologist treating a teenager who had been a victim of child-trafficking from England to the USA, as part of the child-pornography trade. Children in that "commune" were coerced to participate in shocking sado-masochistic actions for a backstreet video industry. But the production company also served as a "front" for a culture of unimaginable sexual exploitation. It was not the victim's PTSD that posed the dominant problem for the therapist (and the entire psychiatric unit), but, rather, the patient's unprovoked emotional outbursts, distrust, manipulations, and other trauma re-enactment dramas that she played out on the unit—including an incident where she threw a chair through the fifth floor window, jumped out of the window, and hung from the parapet until the therapist and two patients rescued her. But several staff sustained quite serious injuries and her therapist required a "prolonged leave of absence."

I use this example to illustrate how Complex Type II Traumas compounded by atrocity participation possibly represent the greatest therapeutic challenge in psychiatry today. In Chapter 1, I identified AXIS II Personality Disorders, such as "Borderline Personality," as the extreme outcome of Type II Traumas.

In my own trauma groups, I have several patients with extremely severe symptoms, and will review the therapeutic modalities that I use below, based on educational workshops adopted by the New York Office of Mental Health.

In summary to this point, the salient differences between Type I and Type II Traumas is that victims of severe Type I Trauma exhibit an acute state of overarousal, distressing recollections, and flight. In contrast, victims of Type II Trauma usually exhibit a set of complex characterological changes that may be quite subtle, with symptoms expressing themselves more evasively, and over a longer or delayed period of time. Type II symptoms also include a variety of personality deficiencies that are sometimes understated and misunderstood by mental health professionals unfamiliar with the basic concepts of healthy self-function. The case I described above of child-slavery in the pornography industry is exceptional in the voracity of personality disturbance suffered by the victim. Such victims will understandably require an expanded set of therapeutic strategies to recover.

General Principles of Trauma Recovery

The degree to which an individual will recover from psychological trauma depends on several factors, including the victim's age, the severity of the trauma, and the speed and effectiveness of their rescue. Trauma survivors immediately placed in a safe environment, especially those united with a familiar or empathic person, are more likely to recover using their own healthy cognitive and emotional resilience. These survivors may also be more effective in mobilizing external resources, such as friends, pastors, or therapists.

Natural Recovery ("Habituation") and Type I Trauma

Most individuals who suffer stress-related symptoms following a single trauma, even after an event that was horrific or life threatening, will experience a natural resolution of symptoms over days or weeks—*even without treatment*. This is a result of what is termed *"habituation."* At a biological level, this recovery occurs because the Hypothalamic-Pituitary-Adrenal Axis is able to "switch off" its stress response once the source of danger has been removed.

After victims are convinced that the state of danger has subsided, they experience a gradual lessening of their sense of turmoil and distress, and begin to make sense of their experience. The majority of survivors of an acute trauma will be able to resume their usual routines within a few hours or days, unfettered by residual fear.

Nevertheless, I have found that such individuals, even without treatment, benefit from empathic social bonding and informal discussions with friends or colleagues at the workplace. The capacity to self-reflect and reactivate the good memories of positive relationships acquired during childhood is healthy, and used by victims with effective survival skills.

In addition, society has a way of healing itself when under attack by turning to communal bonding behaviors. This function appears to be built-in, even among *non-primates*, where animals in the wild show protective behaviors toward a wounded communal member.

I would like to add here that one does not need to be a therapist to have the gift and ability to heal. Healing also occurs through natural empathic social bonding. Assault victims feel relieved by sharing their story with closely trusted friends and family. Many victims have told stories about how even casual encounters with acquaintances had a therapeutic effect in lessening their sense of fright following an assault.

In contrast, the breakdown of communication networks, assassination of journalists and outspoken leaders, and the disappearance of community members in a terrorized environment elevate stress levels throughout the community. This compounding effect of trauma prohibits self-healing and will require a comprehensive approach to recovery that includes rapid and effective intervention by community resources or other external rescue agents. Healthy survivors have developed adaptive coping skills that facilitate access to external resources that may prevent the onset of either class of trauma syndrome.

What I have described above refers to situations where individuals' adaptive responses are sufficient for recovery and require little, if any, limited formal treatment interventions. Healthy self-caretaking functions include relaxing, taking time off, dedicating more time to religion or recreation, playing sports, developing a hobby, and other recreational activities such as soothing music, painting, reading, and gardening. These activities and practices are effective when trauma symptoms are limited in time and scope.

Recovery from Acute Stress (Type I Trauma) Symptoms

If you have experienced an unexpected physical or sexual assault, then you may be one of the 90 percent of victims who experience significant emotional distress during the ensuing days or even weeks. Nevertheless, in certain highly traumatized populations, numerous studies indicate that after 12 weeks there is a 30 percent chance you will remain significantly distressed.

Children who are assaulted or abused are even more prone to experiencing terror, fear, and turmoil in the days and weeks following prolonged or repeated trauma. In more vulnerable subjects this can occur even after a single severe trauma occurrence.

Rescue, resources, and surrogate caretaking are areas that are vital to the recovery process. Communication with loved ones has been shown to be both the most common and psychologically reassuring behavior among survivors of a terrorist attack.

Failing to establish contact with one's loved ones leads to prolonged stress-activation. The public should be forewarned to establish early contact with family and friends following any disaster. After a personal assault, a victim is advised to share at least something about his or her experience with someone who is close and has empathic qualities. This "ventilation" is crucial for psychological relief.

When physical rescue from danger is delayed, or there is some form of caretaker failure, this also intensifies the severity and duration of stress symptoms. From a biological perspective, the quicker one can contain the acute stress response the better the prognosis.

The eventual goal of recovery is to pull together all the chaotic trauma fragments and establish a trauma narrative that can be safely located in the past and comfortably recalled in the present without causing undue distress.

Therapy for Victims with PTSD

When a person's coping skills or defenses are overwhelmed, however, the ensuing symptoms of PTSD (or of Complex Trauma) have to be identified, and victims should consider a variety of more formal therapies. Following an assault, the first priority is to find safety, calmness, and be focused and anchored in the present.

For patients with either Acute Stress Disorder or PTSD, the most effective treatments are those described in the discussion of Behavior Exposure Therapy and medications, which should be used selectively. The goal for the victim is to reduce the level of stress and arousal and overcome avoidant behaviors.

In therapy, you-as-victim will be required to confront your traumas within *your* comfort zone, so that you can then "move forward" without apprehension, fear of traumatic memory images, or entrapment in a constant state of psychological "fright or flight." Ultimately, you will construct a coherent *"trauma narrative"* (or story of what happened and what it means to you) that you can comfortably confront and then put to rest. You must be willing to confront the pain about what happened to you.

Prior to recovery, the traumatic events may be scrambled in your mind, rendering you vulnerable to any trauma-triggers or raw trauma fragments that will be triggered time and again, unleashing the same pattern of fright and arousal. Having identified that you were a victim, you will then need to recall the details to which you can give a chronology and context. You will then be able to patch together the unfortunate trauma-related events that occurred at some critical point in your life.

In this process, you can invoke *dual awareness* (discussed above), which requires the strength to face the *past* while feeling empowered and secure in the *present*. You will need empathic support as you confront the pain about what happened to you.

In addition, this process of narration, recognition, and awareness should be done incrementally, within the mutual discretion of your unique therapeutic relationship. In time you will need to widen your horizon of painful exposures but, simultaneously, be "anchored," calm, mindful, and emotionally supported.

Until that point, your repression of traumatic material and avoidance of trauma-reminders caused your retreat from spontaneous engagement in the present. Sealing off your pain for so long may deprive you of ever living your life fully in the present. Now it is time for you to leave your damaged past and move on, engaging each new situation without feeling compromised or intimidated.

The mechanisms of natural recovery from trauma are strong in humans, as discussed above, and lead to gradual dissipation of acute traumatic symptoms, including those early symptoms that resemble PTSD. However, among those victims who show severe and persistent symptoms and are unable to recover for a variety of reasons, about 30 percent develop PTSD.

Chronic unresolved trauma may also lead to structural personality deficits, where victims continue indefinitely to feel deficient and act in a self-defeating way, in perpetual trauma re-enactments.

A Case Example: In the ensuing turmoil of a rape or terrorist attack, help and rescue may be delayed. Conventional safe havens may be demolished, and individuals are left with nothing more than *themselves*. Those who are older or more resilient may be able to remain calm, focused, and even capable of heroic acts of altruism. Victims who are young or otherwise more helpless may be totally overwhelmed by a trauma and "*lose themselves*."

Psychiatrists refer to this phenomenon as "dissociation," and it is the cornerstone of Acute Stress Disorder. In Chapter 1, I described a severe case of Acute Stress Disorder in a victim of the first tower of the World Trade Center hit by the terrorists on 9/11. She exhibited the most extreme form of dissociative symptoms I had ever seen; the victim was so fixated on the visual imagery of the trauma that the "present moment" in time did not exist. I was sitting in a "place" with a victim who was totally immersed in a continuous reality of smoldering death.

For such catastrophic reactions, my priority was to attempt to lessen the degree of fright and then re-anchor her into the safety of the present. To accomplish this, I chose not to admit her to a noisy, hectic psychiatric unit. This would have been more likely to increase her sense of confusion, fear, and turmoil. Instead, I recommended that her mother take her home to her own room, dim the lights, play soft music that she liked, and take off several days from work to be at her side. This approach would also serve the goal of lessening the victim's exposure to other sources of stimulation that could result in further physiologic overarousal. She needed to be shielded from any external intrusions, such as TV and even the telephone.

Since she was in a perpetual state of heightened arousal (illustrated by the pacing, moaning, and inability to sleep), I prescribed minor tranquillizers to lower her arousal levels. I encouraged her mother to gently engage her, periodically, with words of comfort and reassurance.

The patient emerged from her dissociative state gradually over about 72 hours. Since survivors with extreme dissociative symptoms are much more likely to develop PTSD, I referred her to our Anxiety Clinic (where we were treating other victims of the World Trade Center terrorist attacks). She then underwent a successful six-week course of twice weekly Narrative Therapy.

Types of Therapies for Victims with Type II Trauma

In order to overcome this multiplicity of challenges, a survivor cannot be expected to follow a generic self-help manual. Behavioral Exposure Therapy doesn't attempt to address the spectrum of symptoms found in Type II or Complex Trauma. Therapists in the field of Self Psychology, Psychodynamic Therapy, or Cognitive Dialectic Behavior Therapy could resolve these issues, provided that the core principals of trauma recovery are followed.

In Complex Trauma, for instance, interpersonal issues confound the treatment, since "trauma re-enactment" is a cardinal symptom. Therapists dealing with victims who try to co-opt them into trauma re-enactment are not always capable of showing these skills, which are emphasized more in the Schools of Object Relations, Self-Psychology, and even traditional Psychodynamic Therapy.

Other victims feel forced (in order to remain functional) to "seal off" their traumatic events, pretending that they never happened. This is even more likely in victims conflicted by a sense of loyalty towards someone close who has traumatized them. The love-hate ambivalence toward abusers causes a confusion, which can also lead to avoidance of therapy. A trauma therapist will attempt to identify all of the issues that have kept the victim resistant to confronting their role as victim.

Victims who remained in any form of prolonged "captivity" may also have suppressed any attempt of discovering their sense of autonomy, including victims of childhood or spousal abuse and political prisoners. Many of them live lives burdened by servitude. For them to recover from this suppression of self-function, they will have to discover their "surrendered identity." These victims have tenuous belief-systems. Some of them may have pathologically identified with their captors' propaganda template. During their state of captivity, these victims became sympathetic to their captors who kept them alive. This phenomenon is what I previously referred to as the Stockholm Syndrome.

Marylene Cloitre describes the challenge of working with traumatic memories. In cases of Complex Trauma, however, specialists prefer to use *emotional regulation techniques* and *cognitive strategies* prior to commencing the "narrative" phase of therapy. Marsha Linehan and Marylene Cloitre have published widely on this subject and I presented some of these techniques at a recent meeting of the American Psychiatric Association.

The first challenge is to identify whether you belong to that group of more severely traumatized victims. If so, you will first need to be prepped on how to deal with emotions unleashed by "trauma reactivation." Failing this precaution, you may simply be overwhelmed with memories and emotions that may even *re-traumatize* you.

Unlearning Fear (or Deconditioning)

Anyone who is traumatized will experience some form of unpleasant emotion, be it fear, shame, or anger. An *"unlearned" emotion,* such as fear, is the title that therapists give to describe a person's basic, first-response to a negative stimulus, such as pain, as well as to frightening visual imagery or the sight, sound, or smell of a predator. When a painful stimulus is *paired* in time with a *neutral* stimulus, then pairing or association can take place, so the innately harmless associations come to elicit the same fear response.

This phenomenon is known as *fear conditioning*, and it applies to all primates. It has even been demonstrated in experiments with rodents. If an animal receives a foot shock, for example, it will subsequently show a similar fear response when it is returned to the same environment—even without a receiving a foot shock. This is called a *conditioned fear response*. Furthermore, this response becomes genetically encoded in those cells of the animal that are responsible for memory and fearful emotions and behaviors. This is adaptive, however, since it serves a protective function: The brain needs to learn what is dangerous in order to recognize and respond to danger.

That is how the *fear circuitry* in a human being serves an adaptive function: If you were assaulted, for example, you may initially have symptoms of worry and apprehension for the first few days, but then these symptoms subside. The same fear-response may be "triggered" in the future, however, if you recognize that this was exactly the same place where the original assault occurred. In this instance, we say that you have become *contextually conditioned.*

The Scope of Fear Triggers

Some PTSD victims have a narrow field of fear triggers while others have a wide field. This factor—the "scope of the field"—refers to whether or not you will able to contain the cascade of fear when you are re-exposed to your fear-triggers. Some victims may re-experience stress symptoms only when shown pictures, movies, or other imagery of the event, i.e., they have been contextually conditioned by visual cues, while others may be sensitive to sound, smell, or other sensory cues. More vulnerable victims may be sensitized to a wider field of secondary and tertiary associations. This sensitivity can become disabling to the extent that the survivor enters into a constant state of vigilance.

Treatment should be considered when the victim continues to experience distress, engages in avoidance behaviors for weeks after the event, or has heightened apprehension triggered by a wide range of trauma reminders.

Therapeutic Strategies for Alleviating Fear and Arousal

What is unique about humans is not only that we can examine our thoughts and emotions, but also that we can understand and change our responses to stress. A Vietnam veteran, for instance, can tell himself at a July Fourth fireworks parade that he is "safe in New York and no longer in a combat situation." He can further explain to himself that the firecrackers are merely "fear-triggers" that remind him of traumatic recollections of being under attack when he experienced fright and horror.

When a victim uses these strategies to prevent the fear cascade of PTSD, he is applying a cognitive strategy in recovery, i.e., a strategy that involves all the normal functions associated with our thoughts and mental processes. This practice is one of the essential elements of Cognitive Therapy, which is discussed more fully below. While fear responses are common in most individuals following trauma, if your fear lingers in the absence of any external danger, you may need to learn such recovery techniques.

Many victims exposed to constant danger without adequate respite, such as victims of spousal abuse, continue to live life as if they are in a "war zone." They exist in an "over-arousal" realm of PTSD, in which even seemingly harmless triggers cause them to experience apprehension, fright—even panic—and the wish to flee.

Therapists refer to such fear-conditioned victims as "adrenaline junkies," meaning they have become permanently conditioned to living in a fear-mode. These survivors are stuck in the trauma of the past, unable to engage the present in either a spontaneous or gratifying way. In such cases, the principal element of therapy is to re-expose the victim to the conditioned fear stimulus and, at the same time, to pair the "fear trigger" experience with something safe or pleasurable. While the original trauma usually occurred when the victim was unprepared and vulnerable, the goal of therapeutic unlearning of the fear is to enable the victim to establish a safe-haven from which he or she can revisit the recollection of the traumatic experience with the support of a "coach" (such as a professional therapist) who provides emotional support, strategic advice, and immediate rescue functions.

The therapeutic components involved in *unlearning fear* include the following:

- Recognizing the nature of the fear responses in your body
- Accepting the symptoms as an opportunity to heal
- Identifying what triggers your fear-response
- Confronting your inaccurate perceptions of danger
- Attempting to convince yourself that you are safe in the present and that the trauma occurred in the past
- Knowing how to anchor yourself in the present during a fear-response

As regards "anchoring skills," you can practice exercises to develop them. The goal is to feel comfortable in the moment by paying attention to relaxing, "floating," and breathing gently, among other things. In general, to develop "anchoring" you should:

- Engage in any activity that soothes you, such as music, meditation, painting, writing, etc.
- Begin to reclaim your life by increasing your social involvement
- Give yourself credit each time you succeed in overcoming a fear

Case Study of Fear Extinction: The following is an example of fear extinction drawn from my professional practice, which occurred when I was treating the 11 Hassidic students who survived the highly publicized "Brooklyn Bridge shooting." The final and most difficult task of this therapeutic process, which included both anchoring and Cognitive Therapy techniques, was to drive the boys over the Brooklyn Bridge in a van. I must stress here that this was possible for only some of the students after 12 sessions of therapy, during which time they learned a variety of coping strategies (cognitive as well as different relaxation techniques). In keeping with various studies of recovery in PTSD, I identified the students' ability to overcome fear and avoidance of the crime scene as the final objective of successful treatment. During this exercise in fear extinction, the students were encouraged to give each other positive affirmations that were paired with joyful Hassidic music while they drove over the Brooklyn Bridge.

While recovered survivors of trauma, such as these students, develop an emotionally manageable narrative of their trauma experience, one that is abstract and organized into a coherent picture, un-recovered victims of trauma remain struggling with terrifying sensory fragments of a trauma that they never processed and stored.

Dealing with Flashbacks

For "processing and storage" of traumatic memory, individuals need robust Hippocampal function to synthesize their traumatic event. The Hippocampus is a part of the forebrain, located in the median temporal lobe, which belongs to the limbic system and is responsible for memory-linked emotion and the fear context. This synthesis is not possible, however, while victims are in a state of neuro-toxic overarousal. When such overarousal occurs, trauma narratives are not properly consolidated. Instead, frightening memory fragments intrude into consciousness, producing the internal experience known as the "flashback." At times, such demonic visitations can trigger a full "dissociative" state, in which the victim travels back in time to the trauma experience *as if it were happening now*.

The purpose of confronting any traumatic memory or "flashback" is to give you control over the memory on *your* terms. Since traumatic memories are negative and painful, survivors prefer to take flight from both memories and external "triggers" that remind them of any abuse or other personal violations. To some extent, you may succeed in avoiding painful emotions by restricting your engagement with your external and internal worlds. Despite all efforts, however, these recollections usually find a way to push themselves back into consciousness. In fact, these unwanted visitations are mere signals that the trauma is still lingering as "unfinished business."

If you never consciously process the traumatic event and organize your story into an abstract script, then it may continue to persecute you, functioning as a constant threat to your fragile sense of tranquility. Before initiating the goal of confronting these internal demons known as "flashbacks," the therapist has to prepare the victim with cognitive strategies, the most common of which are skills known as "anchoring" and "self-soothing."

Once you are emotionally and consciously anchored in the present, you can gradually gain a sense of knowledge and mastery over your trauma. You may achieve anchoring in a variety of ways discussed above, such as through "mindfulness"—a form of meditative self-awareness (discussed below) and cognitive analysis, which involves the ability to recognize fear triggers and respond in a more effective way. Finally, you will emerge from the sense of being out of control, at the mercy of the trauma.

Therapeutic Trauma Exposure

Parents, therapists, and political leaders need to successfully convince victims that the *world is safe again*. This process is necessary to create a safe holding environment, which will enable the victim to recover through "exposure" therapy via imagery or narration. This protective environment allows for a gradual process of "extinction"—a process of reduced emotional response with repeated exposures to traumatic memories or "triggers" in a safe or supportive setting. Using this method, Edna Foa, an expert on PTSD, has found that patients' repeated trauma narratives become less intense and affect-laden. When patients repeat their trauma narratives again and again, they become much more abstract compared with their prior trauma descriptions, which are initially reported in a dramatic and sensational way. That means that "telling one's story" allows victims to develop a representational form of memory that is more conceptual and analytic, and replaces the earlier trauma memory that was dominated by intense sensory images, thoughts, and feelings.

An additional goal of therapeutic trauma exposure therapy is that *narration* provides the story with a time-line, or chronology, which *anchors* the survivor in the *safety of the present*, and thereby creates a clear distinction and distance from the trauma of the past.

Sometimes trauma survivors avoid the above process and "seal over" their painful experiences. For instance, Holocaust survivors often have a prolonged adaptive period of functioning until they are faced with another traumatic loss or threat. In the long run, most chronic trauma survivors will have some form of re-activation or re-enactment of trauma-induced symptoms when exposed to the triggers that elicit *conditioned fear*.

Only through processing and confronting their painful memories can survivors gain a sense of mastery over them. The failure to do so leaves victims vulnerable to subsequent trauma-triggers, which unleash the fear-cascade. This may result in victims exhibiting excessive social and emotional inhibitions—or avoidance behaviors.

Since therapeutic exposure may backfire if the victim is overly fear-sensitized and lacks sufficient internal coping strategies, clinicians unfamiliar with trauma recovery may recoil at the notion of "revisiting" (via imagery or narration) the traumatic event. The term "exposure therapy" does, to some extent, involve the process of *forcing* clients to "relive" their trauma by repeatedly recalling the horror of their traumatic event in therapy. But, on the other hand, "supportive therapies" that continue to coddle and protect the victim come at the expense of perpetuating a life of external flight, or an inner world devoid of any thoughts or emotions dominated by avoidance defenses.

While the therapist's intuitive feeling may be that this endeavor inflicts pain on their clients, in reality most victims are *relieved* at the opportunity to "ventilate" their trauma in a safe environment.

Identifying if the Therapist Is Right for You

While exposure therapies are useful for trauma victims dealing with simple fear responses, those who have been exposed for a prolonged period of time to interpersonal trauma will need additional strategies to recover. For example, victims of early abuse respond to simple exposure therapy only about 20 percent of the time (see Marylene Cloitre's *Treating Survivors of Child Abuse*). For such patients, the school of Self-Psychology, among others, can become a vital adjunct to Cognitive Therapy.

While Type I Trauma sensitizes the world of the victim to a life dominated by fear, victims of Type II Trauma struggle in a world of servitude and trauma re-enactment.

In the case of severely abused children, for example, the therapist must bring abundant empathic skills and resources into the therapy to compensate for early caretaker failures. These skills and resources are even more critical in cases of Complex Trauma, where lack of trust and deficient self-soothing abilities are major obstacles to recovery.

If you are using or intend to use cognitive analysis to treat Complex Trauma, then this will require that you and your therapist explore and adjust, when necessary, the full spectrum of symptoms described under Complex Trauma, such as feelings of fear, guilt, shame, and being controlled by others. These perceptions do not happen "out of nowhere." They occur as a result of our personal vulnerabilities, which are being generated by specific "triggers."

There is inevitably a sequence, a chain of events that precedes our sensations, thoughts, and interactions, which are harmful. Furthermore, if we probe deeper, we may recognize a pattern. You can learn about how similar triggers elicited negative feelings and unwanted behaviors in you in the past. To do this, you first need to find these triggers. Then, you need to itemize the silent chain of internal responses that precede the maladaptive behavior. You also have to take responsibility for your actions and realize that *you do have the power to interrupt the sequence of events that follow the triggering event.*

As with all trauma victims, survivors of Type II Trauma require treatments by therapists versed in a wide range of skills. If you have experienced sexual abuse or spousal battery, you may have difficulty with trust, emotional regulation, and anger. You may also show a propensity to re-enact your trauma in the therapy.

You, as a trauma client, should establish, therefore, that the therapist has the following skills and capacities:

- The therapist is clearly attentive to your abuse story
- The therapist appears to believe you about what happened
- The therapist tries to understand your feelings
- The therapist is methodical in identifying a list of trauma-triggers
- The therapist accepts you and is not judgmental

The above-mentioned items address some of the benchmarks that would indicate a positive therapeutic process. The following items are some benchmarks of progress in setting therapeutic goals:

- The therapist shows concern for your well-being, so that you feel less isolated and more empowered
- The therapist enables you to learn an array of new and more adaptive responses to threat, e.g., instead of being obedient in relationships, you will become more assertive
- The therapist helps you compile a list of negative emotions, such as fear, anger, or shame, that are triggered in you by everyday experiences
- The therapist helps you identify a list of stress-induced and often self-defeating behaviors

Challenges to the Therapist

In survivors with Type II Trauma, multiple skills on the part of the therapist are of paramount importance to maintain the safety of the therapeutic relationship. For optimal recovery, the therapist should have the following traits and skills:

- Be familiar with trauma-recovery techniques
- Bond well with the victim
- Have the resources to provide some caretaking function
- Be familiar with current techniques to help you identify and manage damaged self-functions
- Have personal, empathic resources to compensate for early caretaking failure
- Know how to avoid being co-opted into the victim's world of trauma re-enactments

The following may be indications that you have the wrong therapist:

- The therapist appears to have difficulty believing your story
- Alternatively, the therapist will question whether you may be exaggerating
- The therapist may minimize your experience
- The therapist may feel uncomfortable with what you are reporting or even try to change the subject
- The therapist may request that you show proof before you make abuse accusations
- The therapist may show discomfort when you report abuse
- The therapist may request that you describe the abuse in detail when you don't feel safe

Example of Problems and Challenges Facing Therapists

All of the above-mentioned behaviors suggest that the therapist is too overwhelmed by the material to organize it for you and provide you with the required coping strategies and support. For instance, in the case I described above involving the childhood victim of captivity and coercion in the pornography trade, the therapist had to deal with several of her *personal* traumas. While trying to rescue the patient from the parapet, she was scratched, which caused a skin laceration. Since the patient tested HIV positive, the therapist underwent mandatory AZT therapy. The medication caused nausea, preventing her from being fully productive. The hospital identified the event as being "sentinel," i.e., an unexpected occurrence that involved the risk of death or serious physical or psychological injury. This situation required immediate investigation at an executive level. Several administrative meetings were held to review the therapist's progress notes. The therapist was interrogated about any "triggers" that should have been identified to preempt the serious suicide attempt. Needless to say, the therapist (a "psych" intern) felt that *she* was on trial. As her supervisor, it was obvious to me that the therapist needed her own supportive therapy and time off, as she began to show signs of a "Stress Related Disorder."

I mention this case in order to illustrate the challenge facing therapists dealing with clients who have suffered serious childhood abuse. The victim suffered from a combination of PTSD, Complex Trauma, and severe Borderline Personality Disorder. Her symptoms wreaked havoc on the unit and resulted in multiple high-level administrative meetings, and the therapist's medical "leave of absence." Ultimately, multiple health care professionals also became co-victims of her abuse history.

Psychodynamic Therapy

M. J. Horowitz, the most noted psychoanalytic trauma therapist, has outlined the principles involved in the traditional Psychodynamic Therapy model. An Individual's unresolved trauma will continue to surface in his or her consciousness as "intrusive symptoms," and be defended by denial (repression) until the therapeutic work of trauma resolution is accomplished. The therapist practicing Psychodynamic Therapy will identify and attempt to analyze the victim's defenses and, in particular, repressive mechanisms utilized to defend the ego against traumatic memories.

Abuse victims have often been so demeaned, their feelings invalidated, their sensitivities dismissed, and their pride demolished that they lose the ability to develop, let alone defend, any sense of "personal rights." Their trauma symptoms may be missed for several reasons, such as when they experience post-traumatic amnesia. As a result of a defensive process of "repression" or "dissociation," they may have no recollection of the abuse that occurred. Another reason abuse is missed is that victims may engage in a process of "rationalization." Some believe their tormentors were "too kind to have done that to me."

This often happens when the abusers were parents, spouses, or other close family members. These relationships lend themselves to a strong component of loyalty. If you deny that you were a victim of abuse but nevertheless present with symptoms of Complex Trauma, your therapist will seldom recognize your constellation of beliefs, emotions, and behaviors as fitting into an *abuse pattern.* This may be seen in the following case of two sisters, Natalie and Paula:

Natalie was a beautiful young woman who came from a stable upper middle class family. Her parents were graduate students and were very nurturing. She presented at therapy for a recurrent pattern of having relationships with men below her educational and social level. She was very innocent, easily swept off her feet, and then emotionally abused until her friends or parents rescued her. She had a sister, Paula, who was 14 months her senior. Paula went into therapy for feeling guilty that everything was going right in her life while her younger sister, Natalie, was stuck in this pattern of abuse and misery.

Paula admitted that when Natalie was born, she felt as if the new baby had taken away her parents. "I hated her so that I tortured her continuously," she said. Paula continued: "She was so good that she always defended me. She just wanted to be my friend." But at the time, Paula's jealousy could not be contained since she felt that her infantile needs had been "stolen away from me."

After Paula had learned to forgive herself (by later understanding that her sibling-envy was understandable), she approached her younger sister. "You should know about what happened." Natalie was then able to utilize this information in her own struggle to free herself from re-enacting this trauma dynamic.

In the above-mentioned case, the victim, Natalie, was deprived of the opportunity to recognize that her pattern of denying and rationalizing the behavior of her aggressor, Paula, contributed to her pattern of re-enacting her abuse schema. When Natalie's therapist discovered that she had been abused as a child by an older sibling, it allowed the therapist to introduce a *trauma recovery model.*

Self-Psychology in Healing

Some victims need a period of recovery before they can address their trauma. The psychological theorist Heinz Kohut emphasizes that, once the self is damaged, healing cannot take place through interpretation alone, but, rather, requires a healing interpersonal relationship.

The school of Self-Psychology insists that healing can only occur through a process of *empathic sharing* between the therapist and the victim. Until this occurs, abuse-victims may be weary and guarded, reluctant to share their horrors with anyone. During professional training, the school of Self-Psychology develops a skillset in therapists who have a positive propensity to empathic healing based on their own innate sensitivity to others. Traumatized patients sense that their therapists have harnessed their empathy into a didactic set of skills.

As an authentic patient-therapist relationship develops, the victim begins to feel safe. Instead of remaining in the traumatized state of fear or emotional isolation, something resembling "good parenting" allows victims to gain a sense of *self*. According to Kohut, for this to occur, the therapist has to allow the patient to dwell in and consolidate the relationship. Eventually the patient "micro-internalizes" the good qualities of the therapist, who functions as a good *"self-object."* This requires the therapist to bring sufficient emotional resources into the relationship to provide a safe "holding" environment. In certain victims of child abuse, this is the therapeutic process that allows recovery from the early *self-object* failures of caretakers. In addition the therapist needs to bring a skill-set to the victim that allows a greater pain tolerance, to help the survivor begin to face the real challenges of everyday life.

Once you-as-the-victim has been soothed, you will need to learn how to *self-soothe*. So, in a sense, the therapist needs to function in the dual capacity of caretaker and instructor. Without this process, the danger exists that the therapeutic relationship will become dominated by powerful emotions of a dependency type. The Psychodynamic school of therapy refers to a victim's regressive state of continued dependence on the "good therapist" as an idealized transference reaction, i.e., the "good parent." Transference refers to the process whereby the patient "transfers" his or her emotional feelings onto the therapist as if the therapist were the patient's *parent* or other primary caretaker. This process also can work in reverse, and so therapists have to be on guard not to become over-engaged in a "counter-transference" reaction by acting out *their* rescue fantasies onto the patient rather than remaining dispassionate and objective during therapeutic sessions. When therapists become drawn into this rescuing role, they may lose their therapeutic efficacy by succumbing to some unfulfilled personal needs.

Trauma Group Therapy

The Group Trauma Recovery Model of therapy can be used either alone or as an adjunct for victims who are engaged in individual therapy. The following assumptions form the philosophical basis of trauma group therapy:

- A group environment is formed consisting of 8 to 12 trauma victims
- Two co-therapists lead the group once to twice weekly over a period of about 8 weeks
- The victim group should be as homogeneous as possible, e.g., groups should distinctly comprise victims of rape, child abuse, spousal abuse, terrorist attacks, and so on
- The common cause of trauma binds the victims, who now recognize that they share a common experience
- During the first stage, trauma-narration is *discouraged* because not all members have yet acquired the coping skills to absorb trauma narrations which trigger their own trauma-recollections
- The prevailing "ground rule" is that each victim's sense of safety has to be respected
- Until all members feel ready to process trauma-laden material, they must learn various coping skills, e.g., boundary-preservation and interpersonal respect; grounding techniques, e.g., controlled breathing; and use of soothing

self–objects, e.g., childhood teddy bears, which reactivate early comforting experiences and feelings of well being. For such victims, the group provides a safe-haven removed from a world dominated by fear triggers.

- The group is taught a vocabulary to label their trauma-symptoms
- If a particular group member feels agitated, then others must obtain verbal permission from that victim to touch him as a form of comforting
- Co-therapists identify distressed victims and try to facilitate the group's capacity to heal
- In providing a safe environment, the therapists function, to some extent, in a caretaking or even parenting role

The therapists meet separately, quite frequently, to assess the progress of the therapeutic group process. They decide at which point the group is ready to enter the "trauma-narrative" phase of therapy. The therapists attempt to educate the trauma-group about how to replace maladaptive feelings and behaviors with more functional behaviors and an enhanced sense of calmness and well being. When good parenting skills are used to create a safe holding environment, then healing takes place via bonding and vicarious learning. Victims feel less isolated with their personal burdens and learn from each other's experiences.

For instance, during the first few weeks following a rape, most victims will have very distressing levels of arousal. But years later, they lack vitality and may appear burned-out and emotionally absent. Follow-up studies of traumatized victims show that most "intrusive" symptoms in the immediate aftermath of a trauma, if untreated, are replaced by numbing, constriction, social avoidance, and physical symptoms over time. This can be prevented by a timely referral to a support group for various trauma populations such as victims of sexual assault.

Neurobiology and Medication in PTSD

An unfortunate reality of PTSD is that it's not "all in the mind." A cascade of physiological changes occurs in PTSD patients indicating multiple changes in their brain functioning. Using new technologies, researchers have been able to demonstrate alterations in PTSD patients' metabolic cell activity and reduced viability in their neuronal cells. Significant biological changes *do*, in fact, occur in the limbic (emotional) areas of the brain at an intracellular level. Standard CAT Scans and MRIs had previously not revealed these disruptions in nerve function. We currently have biological markers that specifically identify the main instigators in the "stress cascade."

Positron Emission Tomography (PET) and functional MRIs are some of the new biological probes used in research centers. The main value of these tests is to teach us about brain function; they are not intended to replace clinical diagnosis by trained psychotherapists. There are far simpler methods than PET or MRIs to make a diagnosis of PTSD. Clinical interviews and trauma scales, such as the CAPS (Clinician-Administered PTSD Scale), are reliable instruments to make a diagnosis of PTSD with over 90 percent accuracy.

What we *have* learned from PET Scans and functional MRIs is that patients with PTSD have heightened states of arousal in the Amygdala—the limbic center for fear activation—which produces

Glucocortisoid Releasing Factor (GRF), glutamate, and dopamine protein molecules. Another brain nucleus is the "Locus Cereleous," located in the "Brain Stem." On command from the Amygdala, it releases another transmitter, nor-epinephrine, which travels down the spinal cord and activates the adrenal glands. These glands, which are the final common pathway in the stress-cascade, produce cortisol and adrenaline—the stress hormones.

The brains of PTSD victims are in a continuous state of simmering activation. When they are exposed to trauma-triggers, their "fear-cascade" becomes further activated with varying voracity, depending on the intensity of the trigger and the victim's vulnerability.

One resolution to this is medication. Articles are published every week in prestigious psychiatric journals that describe the success of new medications for PTSD. In truth, although drugs such as the selective seratonin reuptake inhibitors (SSRIs), mood-stabilizers, and benzodiazepines *do* help relieve some symptoms, they do not cure PTSD.

The rationale behind the use of SSRI drugs is that serotonin in the brain exerts anti-stress effects by blocking dopamine and nor-epinephrine. SSRI drugs increase the amount of serotonin in the brain, which *reduces* both neuro-excitability in the limbic emotional systems and the production of nor-epinephrine in the brain stem. As a result, serotonin gradually switches-down the over-activated fear circuits in trauma-victims with persistent stress symptoms. Notwithstanding some uncomfortable side effects, such as nausea or headache, these drugs are generally safe when properly administered.

Benzodiazepines are "minor-tranquillizers" that exert a calming effect via a different mechanism: These drugs attach to receptors in the brain that cause rapid "hyper-polarization." A brain cell that is "hyper-polarized" is resistant to excitation. Benzodiazepines such as diazepam and alprazolam will blunt the fear-response in anyone exposed to a fear-trigger.

If you have PTSD there is always a temptation to enjoy the buffer offered by a drug that will keep you in an emotional comfort-zone. I have seen PTSD patients in chronic states of over-arousal that cannot "survive" without using benzodiazepines. They are sometimes the only agents that provide chronic trauma victims with temporary relief.

Although many physicians, particularly in the United States, are reluctant to prescribe this class of drugs, benzodiazepines remain the most effective antidote for all forms of anxiety. The reason for this is quite simple: Those areas of the brain involved in fear-activation have innate benzodiazepine (also referred to as GABA receptors). Within minutes of attaching to the receptor site, the drug activates the receptor, serving as a brake-system, which prevents the fear-cascade.

There is considerable risk, however, of developing addiction to benzodiazepines. As long as your PTSD is not resolved, living in stress and fear can hardly compete with the quick relief-effect produced by these drugs. When PTSD victims take benzodiazepines, their dreadful feeling of autonomic arousal and threat is replaced by that of safety and calmness.

I therefore attempt to limit the use of benzodiazepines to managing stress symptoms for the short term while the victim learns to heal using one of the psychotherapies. Psychotherapy also tends to provide better long-term control of symptoms, while benzodiazepines provide only short-term relief.

Some physicians prefer the use of drugs classified as anticonvulsants, such as gabapentin, a drug also prescribed for mood disorders. This drug, like its cousin valproic acid, works by releasing GABA. Unlike diazepam (often referred to by its trade name "valium"), the anticonvulsant mood stabilizers do not attach directly to the GABA receptor to produce immediate relief of fear and arousal. Instead, they increase the body's intrinsic supply of GABA, a process that takes several days. Their advantage is that, in the long run, the mood stabilizers reduce neuronal excitability without the risk of addiction or dependence.

Alcohol acts in the brain in a similar way as benzodiazepines, but is far more toxic to the liver, stomach, and central and peripheral nervous system. Many trauma victims who remain untreated and "unsoothed" (usually war veterans and victims of child abuse) unfortunately turn to street drugs. The drugs most frequently used by PTSD victims in the veteran population are *hydrocodone* and *oxycodone*. These "controlled substances" belong to the *narcotic* class of drugs.

Surprisingly, the reason for these victims seeking narcotics is not to get "high." The Amygdala is saturated with both opioid and benzodiazepine receptors. When benzodiazepines attach to their receptors, traumatized victims feel calmed, as mentioned above. When narcotic drugs attach to their receptors, traumatized victims feel soothed. When PTSD victims take benzodiazepines, their sense of fright is replaced by that of safety; when they take opioids (narcotics), their sense of dysphoria (negative mood state) is replaced by that of euphoria. Opiods mediate the function of feeling soothed.

It is no coincidence that those parts of the brain involved in trauma have unusually high concentrations of both benzodiazepine and opioid receptors. One must assume that these receptors serve as built-in "brake-systems" for the relief of trauma-induced fright and discomfort.

It is quite feasible that both narcotics *and* benzodiazepines cause more *relief* to distressed trauma victims than those drugs physicians prefer to prescribe. Unfortunately, the risk of narcotic-dependence in PTSD limits the value of opioids. Since PTSD symptoms are often chronic, the temptation to self-medicate re-places the hard work of "recovery" involved in psychotherapy. Furthermore, when PTSD becomes compounded by "substance abuse," it places a burden on the therapeutic relationship, since doctors and therapists are always on the alert to avoid "drug-seeking" patients for their own legal protection.

An additional problem posed by both narcotics and alcohol is their detrimental effect on work consistency and family stability. In addition, some PTSD trauma survivors, seeking any desperate at-tempt to self-soothe, turn to *totally inappropriate* drugs such as *cocaine* and *amphetamines.* Instead of providing relief, these drugs usually exacerbate PTSD symptoms because of their *activating* effect on a brain that is already excessively "wired-up."

Managing Complex Trauma: Victims of Extended Interpersonal Abuse

In this section I will try to clarify certain treatment implications that arise for individuals with trauma-generated syndromes that are not yet formally included in the current diagnostic groupings by the American Psychiatric Association. In particular, I will focus on individuals with enduring emotional and cognitive problems and impairments in social functioning and in victims of prolonged in-ter-personal abuse or terror.

The argument in favor of creating a new diagnostic entity for victims of extended inter-personal abuse is compelling. The victim may not suffer from PTSD but is burdened by a lack of sense of agency (i.e., not feeling "in charge"), emotions that are either un-controlled or over-controlled, chronic physical symptoms, frequent re-enactments of their unresolved interpersonal distortions, and an altered way of looking at themselves, relationships, and the world at large.

In confronting and transforming Complex Trauma symptoms and behaviors, the cornerstone of the preparatory stage is for you, the victim, to feel secure enough to examine your trauma-triggers and responses. Learning new ways of thinking, feeling, and behav-ing can only occur in a safe environment. Although I have a favor-able prognosis for some survivors, I have seen many victims of severe and prolonged abuse who continue to struggle with their demons. Success is gauged by every new, adaptive change in the way you engage the world in a more effective, self-actualizing way.

The following list identifies some of the cardinal symptoms of Type II, or Complex, Trauma. Although this topic was discussed in detail in Chapter 1, I will here itemize important self-functions that are targeted for therapy in victims of Complex Trauma:

- Poorly regulated emotions
- An inability to contain emotional outbursts, or, alterna-tively, a shutting-down of emotions
- Lack of skills in self-soothing and emotional regulation
- A deficient sense of autonomy and power-dynamics
- An inability to set or respect boundaries

- A sense of helplessness and isolation
- Altered perceptions of oneself, such as being "damaged" or "contaminated"
- Altered self-schemas that create a mental vulnerability for re-enactment of trauma
- A vulnerability to adopting the perpetrator's belief system
- Structural dissociation, or a split between the victims' "emotional-personality" and "apparent normal personality"

Many victims of chronic abuse find a way to remain "operational," working, and even to show a semblance of social engagement. But their emotional selves are split off and isolated from the world, immune to growth, and defended against any sense of joy or pleasure. Establishing a viable "dialogue" between these two components—the operational and the emotional—and integrating the victim into a "whole" is a challenge (for a good description see the *Haunted Self* by van der Hart et al.). This challenge would also apply to the treatment of "Multiple Personality," one of the most serious Personality Disorders.

Challenges to Regain a Sense of Mastery

The following is a list of challenges, drawn primarily from the Cognitive Therapy model, generated by your personal trauma history that will allow you to regain a sense of mastery over your destiny.

- Establish some awareness of having been a victim
- Make a choice to reclaim your life
- Become ready to examine that you were once damaged
- Admit to feeling angry about being damaged
- Take ownership of your rage against your perpetrator

- Forgive yourself for allowing the traumatic experience to happen
- Be willing to examine the effects of the trauma on relationships with those close to you
- Be willing to examine how being a victim affects your relationship with authority figures
- Be willing to examine whether the secret of your trauma isolates you or makes you feel different
- Understand that, as a victim, you need to rediscover your self-worth despite the damage
- Admit to feeling uncomfortable with yourself
- Learn to identify painful emotions
- Be willing to learn strategies that will no longer allow you to re-enact the victim role
- Identify the symbols and situations that trigger your negative emotions
- Explore all the other emotions that trauma triggers might reactivate, such as fear, anger, shame, helplessness, or disgust
- Examine whether these feelings may have caused you (in the role of victim) to have withdrawn from engaging in any situation where you perceive danger
- Choose to feel safe and comfortable
- Be willing to regain a sense of power over your destiny

As a victim, you may have *allowed* yourself be taken advantage of, but now you need to fashion the template for a new reality, one in which you engage the world feeling safe and confident.

The "Mindfulness Approach"

In victims of chronic Type II Trauma, to avoid excessive exposure to trauma material, it is crucial to educate and guide the victim, using the subject's level of pain tolerance to determine the capacity for further trauma exposure via narration.

First, the victim needs to become armed with the strategies of being an empowered adult living in the present. When confronting the "living" trauma narrative, the victim needs to recognize that the trauma events really occurred in the *past* and have no real existence in the present. This is what is meant by "dual awareness" discussed earlier.

When reactivated, if these trauma-reminders generate heightened arousal, they must be effectively contained. Only then does this practice become constructive and allow the victim to metabolize the traumatic event. For the victim, an ultimate goal is to extinguish the fear component of the trauma narrative. Using the cognitive model, you, as a victim, are encouraged to also examine other psychological and behavioral domains affected by your trauma experience. These will vary from one trauma victim to another.

The practice of meditation can be effective in helping you to live in the present and develop "anchoring" and "mindfulness" skills. Adapting the principals outlined by Marsha Linehan in her *Skills Training Manual*, you may find the following steps helpful: They include being mindful, accepting, observing, describing and participating. For each of these steps, consider the following strategies you can develop:

1. *Being mindful:*
- Do one thing at a time
- Focus your attention on the task at hand
- Avoid becoming distracted

The following synopsis of lessons by the Zen Master Thich Nhat Hanh well illustrates the concept of mindfulness and its relationship to anchoring.

"While washing the dishes one should only be washing the dishes, which means that while washing the dishes one should be completely aware of the fact that one is washing the dishes.

"At first glance, that might seem a little silly: why put so much stress on such a simple thing? But that's precisely the point. The fact that I am standing here, and washing these bowls, is a wondrous reality. I am being completely myself, following my breath, conscious of my presence, and conscious of my thoughts and actions.

"There's no way I can be tossed around mindlessly like a bottle slapped here and there on the waves.

"If while washing dishes, we think only of the cup of tea that awaits us, then hurrying to get the dishes out of the way is as if they were a nuisance. Then we are not washing the dishes to wash the dishes. What's more, we are not alive during the time we are washing the dishes. In fact, if we can't wash the dishes, the chances are we won't be able to drink our tea either. While drinking the cup of tea, we will only be thinking of other things, barely aware of the cup in our hands. Thus we are sucked away into the future, and are incapable of actually living one minute of one's life."

2. *Accepting:*

- Accept what happened as being beyond your control
- Accept yourself but decide to change emotions or behaviors that were harmful
- Practice your skills but don't condemn your failures

3. *Observing*:

- Notice what's happening without getting caught up in the experience
- Let feelings and thoughts come into your mind
- Be like a guard at the gate of your palace
- Control your attention
- Notice what comes through your senses
- Notice what you feel in your body
- Notice your actions
- See how others are reacting
- Don't lose yourself and get caught up in mass hysteria

4. *Describing*:

- Put words on the experience
- When a feeling or thought arises, acknowledge it
- Put a name on your feelings, such as "I am afraid"
- Describe your physical symptoms, such as "my stomach is tightening"
- Remind yourself that it's *your reaction,* without getting caught up in it

5. *Participating*:

- Act intuitively from a position of calmness and wisdom
- Do what is needed in each situation

Changing Interpersonal Schemas in Victims of Type II Trauma

Instead of a spectrum of fear and over-arousal caused by Type I Trauma, "interpersonal schemas" describe trauma-generated feelings about oneself as being vulnerable, powerless, incompetent, and abuse-prone. Predators tend to constellate around people with these schemas and exploit the deficiencies they generate.

In fact, many abuse victims have difficulty freeing themselves from trauma-re-enactments. Its relevance is most manifest in patients suffering from Complex Trauma. Rather, this subject is best addressed using the Cognitive approach of "mindfulness." While rooted in the tradition of Eastern Zen philosophy and meditative techniques, this was innovated by Marsha Linehan for the treatment of borderline patients, most of who were discovered to have histories of child neglect or abuse. It has now been adopted by the school of Cognitive Therapy. Its central element requires the victim to identify emotional and behavioral responses produced by trauma-expectations in relationships, replacing self-destructive behaviors with far more adaptive coping strategies. The state of the *emotional mind* is replaced by the *calm mind* using a variety of meditative techniques. This corresponds to a physiological state of low arousal conducive to restoration of healthy Hippocampal function, which facilitates synthetic learning. In this calm, inner-environment, the therapist has far more leverage in transforming your trauma-generated schemas into healthy, adaptive ones.

Confronting Altered Perceptions of Meaning

The alteration of a victim's belief system is one of the cardinal symptoms of Complex Trauma. Victims of child abuse will need to confront their distorted beliefs about being "bad." Rape victims will need to confront their distorted beliefs about being "contaminated" or "defiled."

This "inversion" of a victim's sense of reality is fundamental to the method used by political tyrants. As illustrated in the classic book *Animal Farm* by George Orwell, the pigs exploit and brainwash the other animals to revere their captors as their saviors. In the same manner, political terrorists change the meaning of words in order to cause ambiguity and confusion between the victim and the criminal. A classic manipulation used by supporters of Islamic terrorists in the media is to emphasize the plight and "humiliation" of terrorists while ignoring the effects of the terrorist acts themselves. Sensing the co-operation of anti-Western media sentiment, terrorists have notoriously "staged" scenes of dead women and children, and even recruited them to function as "martyrs" (another word-perversion).

Another classic example of distorting beliefs and value-systems is the "Stockholm Syndrome." For instance, during the debriefing after American hostages were released by Iran, psychologists were shocked when they discovered a paradoxical positive identification of the victims with their captors.

If you are a victim of any form of Complex Trauma, you will have to "tease-out" fundamental beliefs that have been transformed by the predator. This process is intricate and difficult, and has to unfold as you attempt to "take back" or reclaim your identity. Integral to your sense of identity is the capacity to critically examine the origin and truthfulness of your sense of meaning of the world. You will also need to identify and examine trauma-generated behaviors originating from the maladaptive beliefs. A carry-over effect of your trauma-generated belief may play out in relationships that become tainted and biased. You may need to develop a more adaptive schema based on fair and objective consideration of different meanings. For instance, you may need to convince yourself that you are *not deserving* of being ridiculed, threatened, or insulted.

In political indoctrination, you may need to overcome the fear of thinking differently from what the government tells you, what you read in the newspapers, and what you see on the TV. Always be skeptical of dogma and demagoguery. Search for informational sources that promote critical thought and autonomy. Don't let others think for you.

Finally, new ideas have to be rectified though new behaviors. Authentic beliefs produce behaviors that are more adaptive and self-fulfilling, reflecting a newfound sense of meaning, tolerance and truth. These beliefs can only be nurtured by being empowered in the present. All of these functions require an approach of cognitive mindfulness.

Managing Anger

After a single attack or prolonged period of abuse, you will experience a wide range of emotions. Anger is one of the most powerful emotions, and it is sometimes a healthy signal of imminent danger that elicits in well-adjusted individuals a *fight* response, just as fear elicits a *flight* response. However, if you have experienced a trauma, anger can be maladaptive if it is over-intense, frequent, or out of control.

I would call your ability to manage anger "maladaptive" if you respond to trivial situations with angry outbursts. You may find yourself "out of control," quick to anger, and prone to blow situations out of proportion. Your angry thoughts of revenge may be carried from the *past* and displaced onto others in the *present*. You may later regret that you lost control.

Some survivors of abuse or other trauma may hold onto a lingering hatred and need to retaliate. Victims of abuse usually were unable to ward off their perpetrators. The carry-over effect may cause them to redirect their anger against strangers or even toward themselves. Victims of abuse also are more likely to commit "hate-crimes."

How to Cope with Anger Responses

A strategy I recommend for helping you cope with anger-responses includes the following "dos and don'ts":

- Step inside yourself and see your emotions flaring up inside of you
- Don't allow yourself to get too caught-up in experiences that evoke anger
- Try using anchoring techniques such as checking your posture and controlling your breathing
- Be aware of symptoms such as rapid or chaotic breathing, feeling flushed, or a rapid heart rate, which physiologically signals that you are in a state of psychological over-arousal
- Be like a "guard at the gate," observing without reacting
- Describe to yourself what is occurring *right now*
- Take a non-judgmental view about what is happening to you
- Choose to stay in the reflective role
- Avoid reacting with "knee-jerk" (reflexive) anger
- Don't get caught in the content of your thoughts or situation or succumb to your emotions

- Resolve to seek ways of changing your thoughts, emotions, and behaviors
- Accept that anger-generated responses, when out of control, can hurt yourself and others
- Do what you need to do to handle provocation but in a way that is assertive instead of by "losing it"
- Move on to the next situation at hand; don't get stuck
- Give yourself positive affirmation when you respond more consciously and adaptively to provocation
- Remain with a situation you can deal with constructively and consciously disengage yourself from situations that are likely to trigger uncontrolled anger responses

Emotional Regulation

The goal in *emotional regulation* is to:
- Identify the negative emotion
- Strengthen your capacity to self-soothe
- Strengthen your capacity for dual awareness, that is, to stay in the present and try to tolerate your discomfort while stepping outside of your narrative to become an observer
- Apply new adaptive strategies such as remembering and actualizing your personal "Bill of Rights," which includes such things as having the right to say "no," having the right to have your own opinions, convictions, and value, and having the right to be treated with dignity and respect.
- Allow yourself you to feel your emotion and identify its source (recommended by Marsha Linehan)
- Avoid "shutting down" your emotions elicited by unpleasant triggers

- Pursue valued goals
- Don't feel guilty expressing that you've been wronged
- Take deliberate action without losing control
- Move on; don't get stuck with what's happened
- Seek supports free of demands and emotional blackmail
- Give yourself positive affirmation for new achievements

The Narration Phase of Therapy

Once you have been rescued from any immediate threat, you, as a survivor, need to feel safe and confident enough to understand what happened so that you can "put the matter to rest." This will require successful completion of the *narration* phase—which is the final phase—of Cognitive Therapy.

Prior to this, the survivor may have to master other elements of Cognitive Therapy, such as strengthening self-agency or anger management. This will prepare victims to have "self-help" strategies that will allow them to face trauma-triggers without being overwhelmed by excessive fright. When this is successful, it will enable victims to confront the past as well as the present with a sense of safety and confidence.

However, not all survivors remain sufficiently calm and focused to build a coherent narrative out of their trauma. Many severely traumatized victims may need to learn a variety of new survival-strategies. Most of these belong to the field of Cognitive Therapy.

Biologically, when the emotional (limbic) brain is overly stressed, it becomes overwhelmed with neurotoxic stress hormones. As a consequence, it loses its capacity to perform the multiple complex tasks required to integrate a "trauma-narrative." The strategies proposed by Marylene Cloitre, however, allow an overly-stressed victim to develop a new skill-set that will restore the brain's resilience.

The new approach to trauma recovery will focus on a wide range of target symptoms, which have mushroomed since therapists have recognized the phenomenon of Complex Trauma. This recognition has revealed the entire spectrum of abuse and provided the opportunity to study new treatment modalities for future victims.

Today's target symptoms include, for example, "alterations in relations with others" and "alterations in sense of meaning." The list of target areas is now wide enough to capture conditions such as the "Stockholm Syndrome" where, as previously mentioned, the victim accepts *as his own* a new sense of meaning to life that reflects that of his predator.

Using instruments such as the SIDES, specific deficits in a victim's self-functioning caused by chronic trauma can be measured both prior to and following different interventions.

The strategies of "mindfulness" include those employed to calm yourself (anchoring), as well as those employed as a self-observer in the recovery process.

In this regard, I recommend the techniques that are discussed earlier in this chapter. Traumatized individuals respond to trauma triggers with predictable thoughts, emotions, and behaviors. Any step along the chain of responses becomes a target for new interventions, once it's established that it is trauma-generated.

The most common reactions in victims of Type I Trauma are fright and avoidance. The most common reactions in victims of Type II Trauma are listed as the "cardinal symptoms" by Judith

Herman. They include such core self-functions as loss of sense of capacity, abandonment concerns, and distortions of meaning.

Mindfulness is a slow process of healing through self-soothing and regaining the capacity to confront and transform all of the distortions set in process by your personal trauma narrative.

In contrast to "normal experiences," abuse experiences have a disorganizing effect on neural pathways. Rather than being integrated like healthy experiences, traumatic events remain amorphous, distorted, set apart from dynamic brain function.

The narration of your trauma identifies the source and uncovers the mystery of how you feel and behave in your daily life. It demystifies your otherwise irrational fears and exposes their origin. Identifying and sharing your trauma removes its power. It becomes relocated in the past, no longer hovering as an imminent, frightening threat. "Narration," in Cognitive-Behavior Therapy, requires that you acquire the capacity to master several strategies in stress management. This can be an ongoing challenge, much as staying "clean and sober" is a lifetime challenge for members of Alcoholics Anonymous, which is based on the philosophy of the "Twelve Step" Program.

Please understand that *trauma narration* does not force you to *relive* the past trauma. Rather, it allows you to revisit the past in the safety and companionship of the present while armed with the coping tools of the present. If these conditions are met, you should be able to tell your story and:

- Re-experience your "conditioned fear" without being overwhelmed by it
- Recall and express any other emotions such as shame or guilt without being overwhelmed

- Be angry when remembering how you were betrayed or abandoned by "caretakers" while feeling secure in your present relationships

The first goal involves that you talk about the traumatic experience in order to *expose and confront its fearful elements* and *dissolve its power to elicit fear.*

The second goal is to put the memory into a narrative form with a chronological order. Narratives convey a story about a life that has a past, present, and future. You should learn to create a life story about what happened that both anchors this terrible event clearly in the *past* and anchors yourself in the *present.* Below I provide a repertoire of behaviors that you will find helpful to realize the anchoring process.

The third goal is to create a present safe-haven that frees you from the grip of past traumatic memories. You need to reinforce your playful engagement in present creative living. This could be accomplished through prayer, sport, art, theatre, gardening, music, crafts, joining a gym or yoga class, or attending lectures, among many other possibilities. Through emotionally engaged living, you will create a schema of yourself that is comfortably engaged in the present and have the ability to distinguish your current experience from the traumatic past. Many adults caught in the turmoil of marital abuse were also victims of child abuse. They may be re-enacting their original trauma, which is what victims are apt to do. Before learning techniques of how to calm yourself and avoid trauma-related symptoms, such as fears or flashbacks, this *safe place* will become the springboard from which you can begin to repair.

Dual awareness is another strategy that is vital for recovery from trauma, during the process of creating your trauma narrative. It is a learned strategy that enables you to connect to the present with the firm conviction that "nothing bad is happening to me now."

All survivors have to practice accessing this safe place at will. What works for each individual, however, is different: for some, meditation may be best, for others gardening, for others prayer, and so on.

You can also use various techniques to help *anchor* yourself in the *present*. This is the safety zone in which you can always seek refuge when faced with intolerable visitations of flashbacks or when overcome with fear or anger. It is then possible, once re-anchored in the *safety of the present*, that you can confront your symptoms and look at the trauma *from the past* but within the per-spective *of the present*.

This is where "role-playing" can often be useful. Using the therapist or recovery group as a support, you can try to confront your tormentor, now as a mature adult. Sometimes roles can be switched, where others role-play you as the victim, or you can change the outcome of the script to that of your liking. What this accomplishes is to demystify and disempower the "tyrant," like in "The Wizard of Oz," whom Dorothy confronts as a total sham.

In the world of trauma, however, symptoms can cover a wide spectrum, and recovery has to be guided, at least to some extent, by the victim. I have seen both trainees and non-trauma specialists exacerbate symptoms with premature trauma-exposure. In other words, victims should not be encouraged to revisit the "crime scene" before they are ready.

The newer therapies recognize that the victim *has to* narrate the trauma in order to process the material, but first be assured that you feel sufficiently prepared to do so. In fact, I recommend that victims who remain severely symptomatic be guided by an individual therapist or participate in a group therapy process.

What has emerged in the psychological literature is the value of learning recovery strategies from clinicians who have been trained to use a modified form of cognitive-behavior therapy, and whose skills include use of empathy, knowledge of relationship therapy, and meditation techniques, referred to by some as "mindfulness."

Marylene Cloitre and co-workers developed much of the work done in this field. The objective of this hybrid recovery model is to allow the trauma or abuse survivor to trust and be guided by a therapist.

The first priority is for the victim to develop the capacity to feel safe again. In this process, the therapist must succeed in creating a temporary safe-haven for the victim before sharing survival-strategies.

The second priority is for the therapist to help the victim to self-soothe. This can be done, for example, by following the developmental model proposed in Self-Psychology by Margaret Mahler. Until you, the victim, have the capacity to self-soothe or emotionally self-regulate, you are likely to remain in a state of chronic emotional over-arousal.

The final priority is to let go of your trauma experience and live each day to its fullest.

Chapter 3

CARETAKER ISSUES AFFECTING TRAUMA SYMPTOMS AND THEIR TREATMENT IN CHILDHOOD

Caretaking Function and Failure

I believe that some form of caretaker participation or collusion lies at the core of all abuse. Caretaking goes beyond the bounds of the "delegation of responsibilities." In all communities, it is caretakers who protect and rescue the most vulnerable members of the community and provide the dominant force for "bonding" between and among individuals. This process is true even for animal communities in their natural habitats.

We now know that healthy bonding between mother and child is an ongoing process characterized by distress signals and empathic responses that begin early in life, possibly even within the uterus. It appears that this function was genetically "hard-wired" during the early evolution of communal bonding. "Surrogate caretaking" is found even in non-primate communities.

Most societies also have individuals, organizations, and institutions charged with both identifying abuse and negligence by parents or others and providing back-up rescue functions. Often even anonymous individuals perform acts of heroism and self-sacrifice following an attack on a fellow citizen. We have all read stories about selfless acts of rescue and personal sacrifice in the news media.

A good caretaker is one whose emotions, voice-tone, tactility, and responses show a total congruence with the needs of another or others. Franz Kohut, the founder of the school of "Self Psychology," referred to this function as "empathy," which implies "being with." This trait requires a certain dedication or "generosity of spirit" towards another.

A mother generally exhibits a variety of bonding behaviors that impact her child's sense of self (which ranges from being more or less cohesive), emotional regulation (self-soothing function), and attentional capacities (mindfulness). These self-functions are challenged in individuals when prolonged trauma exposure occurs in adult populations, such as in ethnic cleansings (genocides) and repeated terrorist attacks. If the victims have had the good fortune of healthy early development, however, then they will mobilize internal or external resources to reawaken good "self objects." Using this process, the victims will be able to access those functions of personal agency that are involved in "anchoring" and "self-soothing" when under attack.

I have discussed these processes and functions in chapters 1 and 2, especially as regards the symptoms of psychological trauma that result from acute assaults on individuals and communities. These symptoms, including behaviors, occur in victims whose coping skills are temporarily overwhelmed. In victims whose development was enhanced by good parenting, however, responses to sudden violent attacks are more regulated.

Certain core personality disruptions can burden some victims during their entire lives. They are illustrated through case examples included in the discussion. In its most malignant form, early empathic failure can condemn the survivor to an eternal search for surrogate parenting, which leads to a pathological dependency on external resources.

This dependence might include compulsive self-soothing in the form of addiction, binging, gambling, promiscuity, or other impulsive, self-gratifying behaviors. These syndromes are highly correlated with child abuse and early sexual molestation. The seriousness of these conditions testifies to the importance of early parental bonding and good caretaking.

One finds failure of caretaking in all of the three groups who are discussed in this book, namely, victims of childhood abuse, spousal battery, and political terrorism. When a parent or other caretaker (including a government) fails to protect, or even colludes in some way with a predator, there is some profound dynamic that has gone terribly astray.

Although I recognize that parents are not always the caretakers, I use the word "parenting" to connote something unique that a "good" parent shares emotionally with a child. It may have to do with the unique bond between a parent and child that will play out in the child's feelings and behaviors later in life.

During the first few years of life, effective caretaking is required for the child to develop a crucial set of psychological and emotional assets. The most important of these assets are:

- A "sense of agency," which includes feeling confident and competent in one's "executive functioning."
- The capacity to preserve one's personal belief systems under stress
- A willingness to engage in rescue-seeking behaviors when faced with threat triggers
- The ability to regulate one's emotions

- The ability to engage and disengage in relationships without feeling a major upheaval
- The ability to tolerate psychological pain and continue functioning under conditions of threat

These functions, indeed, become the main target for the predator. Individual and political predators choose methods that challenge our safety assumptions and threaten our autonomy. In situations that involve both domestic abuse and political terror, the predator imposes a dynamic of fear and intimidation on victims, such as by disrupting their access to rescue. Once victims lose their personal agency and beliefs, they may no longer even attempt to mobilize rescue functions.

Abused children show diminished capacity in several of the above-mentioned areas. While *all* trauma groups include some form of *caretaker* failure, when abuse is perpetrated on the young, it is particularly egregious because of its long-term effects on the above-mentioned areas of personality functioning.

Other concepts relevant to early caretaker failure pertain to "trauma schemas" embedded in young victims who grow up to expect abuse-dominated relationships and participate in them later in life.

The Caretaker and the Predator

When attempting to understand psychological trauma experienced by groups such as children and spouses, it is extremely important to focus on the victims' closest relationships. I therefore emphasize the profound implications for victims when the intimate trust between themselves and their caretakers has been betrayed. And I repeatedly address the issue of "caretaker complicity" when describing the dynamic in which the trauma plays out between the victim and "predator," such as an abusive parent or spouse. To convey this dynamic, I have presented anecdotes in this book that reveal the hidden dynamics beneath the events victims describe (their "trauma-narratives"). The anecdotes demonstrate an inextricable complicity between the caretaker and predator in many cases of civilian abuse as well as in acts of political terrorism (discussed in the next two chapters).

In this book, the concept of "caretaker" applies to an individual (e.g., a parent), a civilian organization (e.g., "Child Protective Services"), or a governmental bureau or agency. In many instances, as illustrated in various chapters, the caretaker *becomes* the predator. This happens most often in domestic settings, such as when a parent abuses his or her child, but this situation also occurs in certain instances involving political terrorism. What I encourage the reader to examine, in short, is not only the psychological damage to the victim, but also the relationships between the victim and perpetrator, as well as the too-frequent failures of society to protect its most vulnerable members.

External Resources and the Rescue Function for Victims of Trauma

How does a caretaking agency protect its citizens in a time of crisis? Abusive and neglectful parents lack the empathy or skills to provide this protective function for their children. When parents fail as caretakers, their failure needs to be remedied through effective monitoring and involvement of social agencies. The vignettes presented earlier of the underdressed, anorexic schoolgirl, and the schizophrenic mother who killed her child, demonstrate that the agencies themselves need to be regulated and held accountable.

Information sharing is a critical aspect of social bonding that alleviates fear. People in countries around the world have demonstrated this on a mass scale during times of emergency, such as war and terrorism. Studies have shown, for example, that a very high percentage of New Yorkers, Londoners, and Israelis attempted to make numerous cellphone calls to friends and family in the immediate aftermath of terrorist attacks. In the 2005 London transit attacks, 76 percent of the population attempted to contact familiar others in the immediate terrorist aftermath, to check on their safety. Individuals experiencing mobile phone network failure, which occurred to a greater extent in New York and less so in London, were more likely to experience substantial stress. Maintaining contact with significant others during a traumatic event plays a vital role in preserving psychological cohesion. This highlights the importance of back-up communication networks in anti-terrorist preparedness, since establishing the well-being of family and friends plays such a crucial role in reducing emotional overarousal.

In the 9/11 attacks, the general population was also desperate to be informed about the existence of any ongoing threat, the identity of the perpetrators, and whether the world's "superpower" could quickly contain or eliminate it. There was a surge of nationalism. Within hours the country was addressed by the President of the United States and informed that America had declared war on Al-Qaeda. Within several months, sustained aerial bombings and ground offensives were launched against terrorist training camps. This retaliatory activity served a "containing" function for a damaged "collective ego," which is so crucial in warding off a contagious reaction of dread and chaos.

In general, however, in the immediate aftermath of an attack on an individual or community, most survivors are left in a heightened state of arousal, apprehension, and even confusion. These symptoms will usually dissipate after days or weeks, provided that the "situation on the ground" is stabilized. This consists of appropriate rescue operations and restoration of normal social infrastructure. In order to minimize the impact of trauma, the survivors have to feel the unimpeded ability to travel, communicate with significant others, and have safe access to food, shelter, and medical assistance.

Recent examples of failure to provide such rescue services to civilian populations include the civil war in Darfur, Hurricane Katrina, and the forced evacuation of 10,000 Jewish settlers by the government of Israel. In all of these cases, the trauma of displacement, separation, temporary makeshift accommodation, and inadequate resources may have caused devastating and probably permanent damage to core ego functions, with children bearing the main brunt of this harm. Many of the adverse effects will emerge later in their lives, and in the lives of all such victims—a prediction documented by many long-term studies of the effects of civil wars in, for example, Bosnia and Somalia, as well as the Holocaust. If leadership fails to provide appropriate rescue functions, then trauma symptoms may evolve into one of the more serious syndromes such as Acute Stress Disorder, PTSD or the Complex Trauma Syndrome.

Childhood Abuse

According to federal law, childhood abuse is broadly defined as an act of failure on the part of a parent or caretaker that results in death or serious physical or emotional harm, sexual abuse, or exploitation. It is an act or failure to act that leads to imminent risk or serious harm. At times, a critical failure of caretaker functioning by a parent requires that the child be placed under appropriate government agencies for protection.

Most urban centers are horribly understaffed, underfunded, and poorly staffed to prevent what I believe to be an epidemic of childhood abuse in America. I would, however, qualify this by suggesting that staffing has to be provided by professionals trained and approved in cultural sensitivity. Such professionals, while recruited from the communities they serve, must obviously satisfy national competence guidelines and state and city oversight.

The spectrum of this kind of caretaking ranges from social agencies that protect children from dangerous parents (or adults from predatorial spouses), to local and federal law enforcement agencies that protect civilians from all forms of threat.

In most cases of serious child and spousal abuse leading to serious injury or fatalities, criminal investigators often uncover a trail of warnings and missed opportunities, such as caseworkers not reporting disturbing signs of trauma to their supervisors, or judges allowing felons free access to their victims, even in situations where the predator posed a continuing threat. Such cases force one to assume that the predator can deftly outwit the negligent or inattentive caretaker, reaching the helpless victim without much impediment. I illustrated this situation earlier with the case of vulnerable children who were left alone with a poorly controlled psychotic mother, who had a known history of violence, and abso-lutely no oversight.

The Protective Effect of Early Development on Trauma Responses

Throughout development a child learns to manage external threats by identifying with and modeling the responses of good caretakers. Early in life, your caretaker will function as an external regulator of your stress responses. You are at an advantage if your caretaker identified your stress signals and responded supportively. Over time, children internalize their parents' coping skills. They may, for example, believe that things will turn out all right, confront problems, plan solutions, and seek support when needed; alternatively, they may be pessimistic, avoid problems, not plan solutions, and ignore support when needed. Internalization of coping skills has been found in various studies. For instance, a study of children during the "Battle of Britain" showed that they suffered fewer stress-related symptoms when they remained with a psychologi-cally healthy parent.

If you have suffered an assault or were the victim of abuse you will need to reestablish your sense of safety and well being. Re-covery is determined by several factors, which include those core self-functions acquired during development that endow every indi-vidual with resilience to trauma. The following factors are relevant to the outcome of trauma, either positively or negatively.

- Good empathic early bonding with caretakers, such as parents, will result in a sense of empowerment and the expec-tation for positive resolution, which will "immunize" the emo-tionally well-nourished child against future stress.

- In contrast, early caretaker failure associated with childhood trauma will render the individual more vulnerable to the harmful effects of future trauma. Victims of chronic abuse are prevented from reaching their full sense of autonomy and comfort in a world they experience as being dominated by predators.

The following list addresses other factors that will impact the individual's vulnerability to future trauma:

- The availability of "rescue resources" if you were exposed to trauma for which you required external assistance, including food, shelter, and access to medical care, case-workers, and even legal recourse
- The severity of the trauma event
- The frequency or duration of exposure to early trauma
- The child's unique temperament during childhood development
- The quality of surrogate rescue caretakers, such as extended family or community, to "step-in" when necessary

The Effect of Resource Loss in Childhood

Resources are an important buffer against of all forms of trauma, and their removal is a universal feature of all traumas. Resources might be psychological (e.g., sense of security) or material. Parents, spouses, siblings, and others who provide social support are the most critical resources. Material resources include one's social infrastructure, such as home, food, school, employment, communication systems, medical care, and relevant governmental agencies.

Childhood is a time when the individual is at the mercy of adults, but, ironically, has limited resources to negotiate rescue and recovery operations. The antidote to trauma is rescue. When the victim is not rescued, recovery cannot commence. Resource loss in childhood can be particularly damaging.

Children can grow unimpeded only in a fertile environment, that is, one that provides them consistently with their basic emotional and material necessities. In a climate endowed with an abundance of resources, the child will learn the skills required to negotiate the world. This occurs in the process of modeling and internalizing adaptive life skills from good caretakers. When these resources fail, community or social agencies are required to function in this surrogate role. In the absence of the above-mentioned resources, recovery cannot begin. This leaves the victim continuously vulnerable and helpless, even against minor challenges. The effect of cumulative resource loss is poor acquisition of self-help skills, impaired social-vocational functioning throughout life, and the accumulation of additional interpersonal trauma.

Effects of Unresolved Type II Trauma

If someone close to you abused you, you may struggle over feelings of loyalty towards your perpetrator. You may have suppressed identifying, let alone reporting, the truth about your abuse. But these feelings follow you into adulthood. Clinicians who treat adult survivors of childhood abuse report a diversity of disturbances in the above-mentioned areas of power-dynamics, relationship-schemas, and emotional-regulation.

Trauma victims may try to over-control their emotions. In fact, they may be so emotionally defended that any idea of feeling eludes them. These abuse victims appear constricted or distant. In contrast, there are some who live in a world dominated by fear or rage, which periodically erupts, sometimes without a clear reason.

Some victims may later feel a need to always be the one "in charge" in any relationship. Other victims fall into the opposite role of constant obedience. Many victims of child abuse will be unable to enjoy the dynamic spontaneity of flexible power sharing.

Your trauma may have stripped you of any sense of control over your destiny. You may tend to compensate for this, therefore, by needing to control the lives of others.

If someone you trusted betrayed you, it becomes hard to trust again. As an example, groups who escaped government persecution in their homelands have difficulty trusting officials, government agencies, or even becoming socialized beyond the safe limits of their familiar culture.

Early Childhood Development: The "Good Caretaker" and Self-Soothing

Knowledge of early attachment of infants to their caretakers helps us to understand why failed parenting (caretaking) can have a damaging affect on a child's mood, sense of autonomy, self agency, sense of self, use of defenses, and outlook towards the world.

The innate experience of the human infant is, by general consensus, unorganized and chaotic. His early environment envelops him, and he is only minimally capable of understanding or transforming it.

Freud's approach to developmental maturation was predicated around the sequential unfolding of the libidinal stages. According to Freud, the human's psychological apparatus is organized around the purpose of lowering drives and tensions, with the predominant role of experiencing pleasure. However, in the account of child development from formlessness to a sequential unfolding, differentiation seems to be to be crucial to many developmental theorists.

For an individual to achieve inner well-being, her or she needs a healthy supply of sharing and validation by caregivers. In this regard, the first bonding between parent and child begins in the womb. A child who grows up in a warm, safe, and nurturing environment is going to carry into adulthood a feeling of security, worth, well-being, and optimism. If you received this type of upbringing, then you will feel more confident and empowered as an adult and will be more effective in your interactions at work and in society in general.

As an infant, your "self" was still in an amorphous state; it had no durable sense of structure, could not stand alone, and required the participation of others for you to maintain your sense of well-being, cohesion and constancy. The psychological theorist Heinz Kohut refers to "others"—from the *infant's* perspective—as not yet separate from the latter's "self." In other words, for the infant there is no sharp distinction between the internal world and external world. The infant's internalized experience of the caretaker becomes part of the infant's internal sense of self, which Kohut terms the "self-object."

Kohut's innovative idea of *mirroring* was subsequently adopted by proponents of the theoretical schools known as Object Relations Theory and Self Psychology. Mirroring refers to how your caretaker anticipated and responded to your needs for both love and validation, as well as to your need to separate from them as you grew up. For Kohut, the ideal situation is when a child is born into an empathic, responsive human milieu. He regards relatedness with others to be as essential for psychological survival as oxygen is for one's physical survival. Donald Winnicott, a developmental psychologist who popularized the concept of the "Good Enough Mother," is in agreement with Kohut regarding the observation that "Disorders of the Self are understood as environmental deficiency diseases."

For Margaret Mahler, another influential developmental theorist, the organizing principal of developmental success is based on whether you, as a child, received and were then able to internalize a stable, cohesive sense of yourself while participating in relationships with those "others" (who appeared as "objects") around you. Mature object relationships require the capacities of balancing self-soothing with sharing and being empathic. Her requirements for optimal mothering bear a striking similarity to Winnicott's "Good Enough Mother." In Mahler's framework, the mother has to demonstrate a capacity to "move with the child in order to enhance the successful sense of confident autonomy."

According to Mahler, the failure to adapt to any stress, particularly in the young victim, is the result of the victim failing to receive critical emotional ingredients from his or her mother or other caretakers. *The benchmark of successful development depends on the movement from a symbiotic dependence on the mother to the achievement of a stable individual identity within the world.* Mahler refers to this *process* as the successful "psychological birth" of the child, or "separation-individuation." This requires a gradual back-and-forth process, a kind of "dance," between the parent and child, which is fraught with separation crises.

From about 4 or 5 months until 10 months, the infant's first phase of "separation–individuation" begins with the process of "hatching." This is when your tendency moves away from a preference of attachment to your mother to the newly discovered adventure of outward engagement and self-determination.

Mahler describes this process of movement from symbiosis to independence as the "practicing" sub-phase. It was spawned in you, as it is in all humans, by the dawning of your capacity for locomotion, such as crawling and climbing. This allowed you, as a child, to move some distance away from your mother.

However, your mother's presence was still required as a kind of "home base" to return to for "emotional re-fueling." Mahler refers to this as the "rapprochement" sub-phase of development. During this sub-phase, however, you, like other children, experienced a need for help from the outside in order to consolidate your confidence in this "individuation" process.

The successful process of hatching and re-fueling is what Phyllis Greenacre calls the child's "love affair with the world," as discussed in her article "Early Physical Determinants in the Development of the Sense of Identity," published in the *Journal of the American Psychoanalytic Association*. Until the completion of this stage, your preoccupation with your caretaker (who is usually the mother but could include any caretaker), and her availability for re-fueling, took precedence over your fascination with the larger world.

During this process, "receiving" occurs via the successful "internalization" of the "good caretaker." Resolution of the rapprochement crisis was discussed in 1971 by Mahler as an essential developmental requirement for the prevention of subsequent psychopathology. The same process has been shown by Winnicott, in *The Maturational Process and the Facilitating Environment*, to be critical for the healthy development of limbic structures such as the Hippocampus.

If you were neglected or abused as a child, you may not have had a caretaker to facilitate this entire developmental process.

Abused adults are often the end result of this earlier developmental failure. The capacity to maintain the sense of autonomy and empowerment is needed to ward off the predatorial behaviors of others. If there was a prolonged failure in empathy, your sense of self-deficits may range from shyness and introversion to serious disorders of the self, such as "Borderline Personality," "Antisocial Personality," and "Pathological Narcissism."

These disorders, which are beyond the scope of this book, are listed as "Cluster B Personality Disorders" on Axis II in the DSM-IV, and are covered at length in the classic book edited by James Masterson and Ralph Klein, *Disorders of the Self: New Therapeutic Horizons.*

According to the renowned trauma psychologist Marylene Cloitre, traumatization is not static. If critical psychological and material resources are not replaced, the trauma-survivor's psychological and social function falls victim to the vicissitudes of ordinary life stressors, further stunting the child's physical, psychological, and social growth. (This was discussed earlier, in the Cognitive-Behavioral section in Chapter 2, on recovering from psychological trauma.) Those who were in a prolonged hostage situation, for example, may continue to feel as a victim, for that sense of danger may never fade. The expectation for re-traumatization exceeds the ability to muster feelings of well-being, or mastery. To counter this tendency and meet these children's needs, responsible parents need to demonstrate appropriate emotional empathy.

This concept also applies to babysitters, schools, Day-Care Centers, summer camps, and so on, where caretaking is temporarily delegated to others. It has been well established that inadequately trained or negligent caretakers can psychologically damage children.

The Role of Early Caretaking in Self-Soothing, Affect Modulation, and Emotional Regulation

The role of early caretaking basically lies in the explanation of what happens during a child's early life, when bonding takes place between the child and caretaker(s). The empathy and validation that your parents (or other caretakers) gave you as a child powerfully impacts many domains of your self-functioning.

A child that grows up in a warm, safe, and nurturing environment is going to carry into adulthood a feeling of security, worth, well-being, and optimism. The more you received this type of upbringing, the more confident and empowered you will feel as an adult, and the more effective you will be in your interactions at work and in society at large. This link between childhood socialization and adult functioning is consistent with the organizing principal of psychologist Margaret Mahler's "map of developmental success." It is based on whether a child received, and was able to internalize, a stable, cohesive sense of self through participating in relationships with significant others.

For this to occur, children have to begin to "hold-on" and internalize that sense of safety and well-being they felt when their mothers or primary caretakers were *there*. Although children experience caretakers as "outsiders" or "others," in that they are objectively separate people, they profoundly shape our experience of the world—and of *ourselves*. The most important "others," whom psychologists sometimes refer to in this context as "objects," are, in fact, our "caretakers." Given the close dynamics of such relationships, good caretakers become internalized as good "self-objects." These soothing self-objects later become available for recall during times of trauma. Alternatively, we attach ourselves to surrogate caretakers such as friends, family, or clergy, to re-awaken latent soothing self-objects from childhood.

According to Kohut in *Restoration of the Self*, children *experience* the feeling-states of their self-objects (especially caretakers) as belonging to *themselves*. The parent's or other caretaker's gentleness of touch, tone of voice, mood, empathic responses, and so on, are received by children and largely define how they feel about themselves. If you, therefore, as a child, were soothed by a good self-object, then you will have developed the capacity to self-soothe, both in childhood and later in life, when your mother is not present. This process will determine our capacity to ward off wild fluctuations in emotions under traumatic conditions.

The ability of your caretaker to "mirror" your experience shapes your sense of safety and well-being early in life. If you received good mirroring responses, then your ability to *self*-soothe and maintain an inner sense of cohesion and well-being, even when faced with trauma, will be strong. These self-help skills need to be accessible for "call-up" during any type of crisis, such as loss, separation, or danger, throughout life. The good self object is more easily *rekindled* via bonding with *empathic* others, such as spouses, siblings, friends, chaplains, or therapists, who then function as surrogate good self-objects during times of crisis. A person's ability to self-soothe, therefore, does not easily take place in a vacuum.

For individuals to maintain emotional regulation during times of trauma, their caretaking functions, both external and internal, can be crucial. In Chapter 2, I discussed in detail how several of these primary self-functions, including "self-soothing," "anchoring," "feeling safe," and "sense of agency," are fundamental to self-actualization and contribute to healing.

In order for trauma therapists to function as "hooks" for the projections of traumatized individuals, they need to be genuine, supportive, and empathic. For the healing process to succeed, patients also need to receive (sometimes subliminally) an emotional sense of being "held" or comforted by anyone with whom they are in a healing relationship. This will make it easier for patients to share their stories in the comfort and safety of "someone who is on their side." Gradually patients will be able to internalize this sense of safety they feel with their therapists as becoming part of themselves. If you are a traumatized individual, then the assets of self-soothing will be critical to re-empower you so that you can begin re-engaging your world with a restored sense of personal efficacy.

Chapter 4

ISSUES AFFECTING TRAUMA SYMPTOMS AND THEIR TREATMENT IN SPOUSAL RELATIONSHIPS

Spousal Caretaking

Caretaking between adults in a spousal relationship requires a mutual exchange of empathy. Two equally empowered adults divide and share caretaking activities (unlike the relationship of parents and children). In a spousal relationship, there may be gender-assigned roles, which vary between cultures, but the betrothal oath is traditionally between mutually consenting adults.

A psychologically healthy spousal relationship follows a shifting dynamic of mutually exchanged empathic responses. Each spouse must adapt to maintain his or her conscious presence and emotionally self-regulate under stress for the "greater good." During illness, crises, or failure, spouses compensate for each other by flexibly shifting the dominant caretaking role. A deviation or distortion of spousal caretaking may consist of one partner becoming detached and withholding, verbally disapproving or demeaning, menacing, or even violent.

While none of these patterns are gender-specific, in a heterosexual relationship we typically think of the abused male as one who is "hen-pecked," while we typically associate the female victim with physical battery. While these "stereotypes" may seem akin to "rules," in truth the more vulnerable or trauma-disposed partner becomes the predominant victim.

The reason for this appears to originate in "learned behaviors." Victimized children often either re-enact their trauma by attracting predators or sometimes entrap spouses into their "trauma complexes," thereby turning these innocent "bystanders" into participants in their trauma narratives. These types of outcomes are, of course, among the most extreme deviations from "mutual caretaking."

To recover from your vulnerability to abuse in a relationship, keep the following in mind and, if necessary, learn these skills:

- You have the right to keep others out of your personal space
- You need to say "no" when feeling manipulated, scared, or pressured
- Consider what is good for *you,* not only the other person
- Make wise decisions to ensure there is always an escape route and the immediate availability of rescue resources
- Communicate spousal behaviors you are concerned about to someone you trust
- Don't be passive when you hear your internal safety-alarm
- Don't shut down when you need to mobilize
- Don't escape into your mind when you need to act
- Assert yourself even if the other person acts upset or betrayed
- Enjoy the ability to "take back" your destiny

In addition to simply applying "strategies," you may have many unresolved grievances that you need to address by speaking to someone you trust. That person does not necessarily have to be a therapist; sometimes a friend or pastor can be helpful.

Many people fervently disagree in their opinions about how to deal with betrayal by an individual they trusted, such as a spouse. Some victims choose to forgive while others do not. Each case has to be judged on its own merit.

Forgiveness is stressed in various religions, but it can put an additional burden of guilt on victims. Guilt itself should be recognized, in this context, as a possible ploy used by predators. Sometimes the test is to overcome a belief that appears to have no real merit. *The path to healing is by rejecting beliefs if they are trauma-generated and cause personal distress.* Such beliefs should then be replaced by interpretations "that work" for a particular individual.

Many offenders, moreover, do not deserve forgiveness; and many victims have good reason to believe they can never again trust or reconcile with an abuser, even a parent. After all, how can they forgive for the life that was taken away from them—their own?

I have seen "people of faith" take solace in the belief that the "Heavenly Judge" will ultimately "settle the score." This belief is helpful and certainly more adaptive for victims prone to acting out their anger or becoming immersed in retaliation fantasies. Those preoccupations just take the victims back to the past and obstruct *creative engagement in the present.* Instead, the role of belief might be adaptive when leading to an acceptance that there is a "Judge, and a Day of Judgment." Once this mind-set is adopted, individuals can free themselves from the revenge-seeking impulses that keep them hostage to traumatic memories that belong to the past.

Spousal Abuse

While many of the principals I have already discussed in this book would be put to good use for victims of spousal abuse, I want to highlight here several other distinctive qualities of spousal abuse and their treatment implications.

In a situation where one person in the relationship has been *conditioned* to be afraid and compliant, you could apply the principles of the Cognitive-Behavioral model. Someone who has previously survived childhood abuse may become either the victim or the aggressor in a spousal relationship. In other words, some victims of childhood abuse may act out their rage as predators, or conversely, participate in a narrative where they function like emotional cripples.

This is illustrated in the following story, based on my personal experience. I had a client who was an intelligent underachiever, affable like an oversized puppy, and constantly in search of attention and approval. His petite wife dominated him, however, in a cold, emotionally withholding tyranny. This poor fellow made a serious but unsuccessful suicide attempt. Following this, he became an invalid. After months in the hospital he returned home where he was placed in a "convalescent room." Few friends visited, as his wife had a way of making them feel unwanted. They had no recourse but to call when she was out, as she would hang up on them.

So his original impulse to escape his tormenting wife backfired, rendering him a complete slave.

When your abuser tries to isolate you, brainstorm with allies how to respond by changing the abuse paradigm that maintains the predator within their powerful comfort-zone. This is illustrated in the following story, drawn from my personal, professional experience.

When I was medical director of a community mental health clinic, one of my social workers was trying to free a victim from her husband's abusive behavior. The client's husband was clearly sociopathic, suffering from pathological jealousy, was a stalker, and monitored his wife's calls, friendships, and activities—even her therapy.

Soon he redirected his rage against the therapist. It began with him leaving threatening phone calls on the therapist's voice mail. With time, as he felt a diminished control over his wife, his threats escalated.

Following one therapy session with his wife, the (female) therapist discovered that the husband had slashed the tires of her car. Following another session, he smashed her car windows. The clinical team met and decided to press criminal charges against the husband.

The spouse abuser was soon served with a "protection order" that prohibited him from having any contact whatsoever with either the therapist or her properties. At the judicial hearing, the judge informed him that any violation of the order would result in an automatic one-year jail sentence.

Behind this psychopathic façade, the husband was a respected member of his community. Being a professional, to boot, this outcome would carry not only a certain negative social stigma but also professional disciplinary misconduct charges.

Prior to the divorce hearings, the client-victim remained terrified. Her husband had a high-power attorney and a whole slew of influential letters testifying to his impeccable character. He had done a good job at brainwashing his kids too.

His wife did not believe she could win marital support, let alone child custody. This predator, however, had not factored into his equation that the protection order listing all of his infractions against the therapist would reach the desk of the divorce judge. It is needless to elaborate that the positive outcome of the case was strongly determined by the mobilization of rescue resources.

Cultural Issues Affecting Spousal Abuse During Periods Of Transition

While abuse typically has its roots in the unique personal abuse history of either the abuser or the victim, spousal abuse may be exacerbated during a period of cultural transition. Eastern and Muslim cultures struggle today with the increased exposure of women to Western centers of education where they are taught about the superiority of parity over dominance in relationships.

When this occurs in a pathological setting, the traditional spousal relationship in a culture cannot sustain the traction of a dynamic relationship between equally empowered adults. Cultural tradition dictates that the male abuser makes the rules while the female victim obeys. The abuser is empowered, while the victim is disenfranchised. The abuser expects unconditional respect. In this situation, an unbiased outside observer can see the abuser's unbridled sense of entitlement and the victim's unquestioning servitude.

I have learned about many of these issues first-hand from a colleague who is a psychoanalyst in Cape Town, South Africa. The town has three predominant communities: European, Muslim, and black. Since the fall of Apartheid, he has observed an interesting cultural, economic, and political shift in family dynamics. Improved wealth and political freedom have provided access to higher education for blacks and Muslims. Considering the vast improvement in social parity, young women raised under Muslim tradition are now learning psychology, philosophy, literature, history, and political science at the University of Cape Town, which still meets universal standards of academic excellence.

However, these young, Western-educated women still marry under the Muslim tradition of arranged marriages and role-assignments. My colleague has related various trauma scenarios revolving around a similar theme: An educated, "emancipated" Muslim woman is still expected to be "obedient." Exposure to Western lifestyles and education creates conflicts with traditional roles and expectations. While the Muslim community is struggling to individuate into Western models, old folklore is difficult to shed.

Religious leaders in the Muslim community are afraid of the threat to the continuity of their culture. The impact of a Western-European lifestyle on Islamic values threatens strongly held cultural mores. When culturally established roles, such as male role-dominance, are challenged, this violates male pride.

My colleague described a recurring pattern in marital disputes: If a husband agrees to have a professional involved in his marital or domestic crisis, he will often not enter the professional's office. Should he do so, he is unlikely to accept responsibility, or take ownership for his own behaviors, or acknowledge the existence of conflict, let alone abuse in his relationship.

At the same time, in such a situation, the female victim is in a dilemma: Should she relinquish "who she is" by turning her back on her cultural ancestry in order to survive psychologically?

There is obviously an emerging need to train mental health professionals to recognize and address these cross-cultural issues in countries undergoing socio-cultural transition.

Chapter 5

POLITICAL ISSUES AFFECTING TRAUMA SYMPTOMS AND THEIR TREATMENT

Political Terrorism

The principles that apply to all traumatized populations apply to political trauma. In the event of a sudden, unexpected attack, the primary symptoms victims suffer, as with any Type I Trauma, are hyperarousal, trauma-recollection, and avoidance. Treatments for these symptoms would, therefore, range from social bonding and information sharing to the full exposure therapies described in the treatment of PTSD.

In our modern age of mass media, the dissemination of real-time trauma imagery has allowed vast networks of electronic and print media to bring terrorist atrocities into the traditional safe-havens of our homes. As a result, after 9/11 there was a direct correlation between people's trauma-related symptoms and the amount of TV they watched about the attack. This was particularly apparent for children included in national demographic studies across the USA. Children who were debriefed by their parents, or who had limited, graphic, TV trauma exposure, experienced less distress.

Victims of terror should seek assistance if they continue to suffer from disturbances in sleep and concentration and have excessive worry. Most victims who experience the above-mentioned stress-related symptoms will habituate after a single attack. These stress-induced symptoms should diminish over time in the majority of resilient trauma survivors. A small but significant percentage of such individuals, however, remain in a state of hypervigilance and are distressed by the visitations of traumatic recollections or "flashbacks." Furthermore, in an unconscious attempt to shield themselves against further trauma triggers, such victims often engage in a variety of avoidance behaviors, which in themselves can become quite disabling. If symptoms in traumatized populations are allowed to linger, however, then the victims are prone to a *recurrence* of symptoms when exposed to a new trauma, even after many years. This has been confirmed by several studies of *retraumatized populations*.

If you have significant residual symptoms of Type I Trauma, therefore, such as PTSD, you will benefit from the trauma-recovery interventions described preciously in this book. The prevailing professional consensus is a preference for one of the exposure therapy techniques.

However, when political terrorism takes the form of prolonged captivity, governmental tyranny, and other prolonged forms of collective assault and deprivation, including victims of kidnappings, maltreated hostages, and survivors of ethnic cleansing or genocide, the trauma will be Type II, or "Complex." These Type II Trauma victims suffer from a wide array of symptoms that extends well beyond that of "fear-sensitization," which I described in detail in Chapter 1, on Complex Trauma.

Within a political context, this type of trauma is usually confounded to some extent by both caretaker failure or betrayal and the removal of traditional safety barriers that constitute the safe "holding environment." One can compare this maltreatment to parental abuse, except that it occurs at a collective level, where the victims are civilian groups targeted because of their religion, ethnicity, or political beliefs.

The strategy of political terrorism has many components. The goal of all terrorism is to achieve dominance over one's victims via physical violation, emotional upheaval, or control over the victims' thinking, as we see in the "Stockholm Syndrome" or members of a cult who have lost their autonomy and ability to think critically. All of this becomes possible once the predator has instilled in the victim a pervasive sense of fear, dread, and terror.

All democracies are jeopardized when governments diminish their threat-perception toward terrorists and their sponsors. Following the 9/11 attacks, multiple system failures were subsequently exposed. The legal prohibitions embedded in civil right laws provided an ideal safe haven for terrorists to travel freely, hide their identities, and transfer money using "front" groups. When a free society experiences such a breach of national security, a serious review of its fundamental privileges has to be re-examined. Similarly, all democracies have to share intelligence information in order to protect global security.

We saw during the Cold War how the Soviet Union succeeded in intimidating, suppressing, and usurping the national spirit of its satellite states, such as Czechoslovakia, Hungary, East Germany, Poland, and the Baltic states.

Caretaking and Its Role in National Security and Political Terrorism

Terrorism includes any willful, politically motivated actions against non-combatant citizens. I would also include in this category any tyrannical rule by governments that forcefully impose their ideologies on civilian society. In certain traumatized adult civilian groups, the individuals' self-functions have become shattered as a result of caretaker failure, in a fashion similar to that seen in early childhood abuse. These traumatized groups include victims of genocide, tortured hostages, mistreated war prisoners, and populations living under "continuous threat."

Consistent with the framework of this book, I conceive of political terrorism as divided into two broad categories: single-incident attacks, e.g., the 9/11 attack on the Twin Towers, and prolonged or continuous attacks, e.g., between the Palestinians and Israelis. This dichotomy parallels that of trauma victims into those whose trauma results from a single assault and those whose trauma results from prolonged abuse. In these two groups, both the victims' experiences and the caretaker's complicity can, and often does, differ.

Just as adults take care of children, governments are expected to take care of their civilians. In legitimate democracies, protection is bestowed as a right on all citizens, irrespective of their gender, color, ethnicity, religion, sexual orientation, or political persuasion.

When governments perpetrate or collude in unlawful intimidation, isolation, deprivation, or punishment of their own (or neighboring) citizens, this is analogous—on a collective level—to the punitive patterns shown by child abusers. In the case of government, the caretaker has transformed its caretaking role into a fear-dominated, restrictive, or punitive dynamic. This form of tyrannical leadership not only replaces an entire society's sense of well-being with that of fear and intimidation, but can demoralize the hopes and aspirations of entire nations. During the Cold War, countries under Soviet rule lost much of their national identity. This form of social abuse carried out on such a grand scale was integral to Stalin's doctrine of intimidation and conquest. One needs to look no further than the former "East Germany," which functioned as the embodiment of Soviet-style militarism and repression from 1945 until 1989. After the fall of Communism, the Free World rejoiced when countries such as Czechoslovakia and Hungary were finally able to reclaim their own national identity. Such epic moments that celebrate freedom over suppression occur whenever a victim is rescued.

After the world has witnessed the toll of tyranny on many national populations for decades, one would expect a renewed commitment of *all* governments to work co-operatively against all forms of tyranny or terrorism and their sponsors. It is a terrible misfortune that the U.N. has abdicated its caretaking role by tacitly colluding with rogue states and terrorists. A caretaker-turned-accomplice played out in the global arena is the most pernicious form of betrayal to all of civilization. When global caretaking ceases, it emboldens and empowers our enemies, making the world *more dangerous*.

The Phenomenon of Enduring Political Terror

Most westerners still enjoy the liberty to express their opinions (even political dissent), without terrible consequences. However, there are countries where public criticism of the government can lead to terrible repercussions. These can range from losing one's job to being imprisoned or even assassinated. Examples of countries that regularly engage in state-supported human rights violations are China, North Korea, and Russia, among many others.

The function of democracy is to protect citizens of all faiths and ideologies. Democracies have a responsibility to protect each other's sovereignty. It is quite tragic, therefore, how caretaker failure in some countries has allowed terrorists and their sympathizers to exploit the democratic privileges of the West and incite racial and ethnic prejudice which, as we know, is the precursor of hate crimes. All democracies are jeopardized when governments diminish their threat-perception toward terrorists and their sponsors.

Prior to 9/11, there were multiple system failures that were subsequently exposed. The legal prohibitions and civil right laws provided an ideal safe haven for terrorists to travel freely, hide their identities, and transfer money, using front groups. When a free society experiences such a breach of national security, then a serious review of its fundamental privileges has to be re-examined.

From a trauma perspective there are studies that show a very high prevalence of PTSD among Bosnian, Somali, and Cambodians refugees, as well as other populations exposed to civil war and ethnic cleansing. In fact, the civil war in Bosnia can be used as a model to study the outcome of the effects of governmental failure in the face of international apathy. According to Nazeda Sajak, who studied the effects of civil war in Bosnia and Herzegovina in 1998, there is a 42 percent lifetime prevalence of PTSD among survivors in those regions. About one third of the population became displaced.

The decimating effect of a failed governmental caretaking function resulted in a compounding effect of prolonged war-related exposure, daily security threats, and other adversities that wreaked havoc among the populace. The destruction of the country's social infrastructure (which I've referred to as the "holding environment") exposed civilian victims to the compounding effects of many adverse elements. In her unique study, Sajak found a high correlation between the number of adversities listed below and the overall risk of people developing PTSD.

- Death or disappearance of wage-earners created socio-economic ruin of family structures
- Death or disappearance of a loved one lead to bereavement
- Civilians lived in a constant state of threat to their personal safety
- There was a high exposure to civil violence
- Family members suffered personal injury
- Family members were separated
- Living conditions deteriorated (including inadequate access to necessities such as food and medical care)

In some countries where terrorism has occurred, the governments have, indeed, "stepped up to the plate" and emphatically established their caretaker function. Peter Curran and Paul Miller, for example, who studied the effect of terrorism during the civil war in Northern Ireland over a 17-year period, showed how the British Government unequivocally asserted its caretaker role in Northern Ireland during an extended civil war. Through successful use of intelligence, the authorities apprehended and prosecuted IRA terrorists. As a result, their attacks became more sporadic and never again threatened to disrupt the civilian infrastructure. Vital *resources* were preserved, including access to food, shelter, medical care, and safe travel to schools and jobs. Consequently, the occurrence of stress-related symptoms in the civilian population was only very mildly elevated.

Resources and Political Terrorism

The manipulation of resources by terrorists becomes a powerful tool in controlling the lives of the victims, for example, by deliberately withholding or removing resources. Their motives range from indifference to corruption to deliberate acts of collective punishment. Such manipulation has the effect of forcing populations into submission or, when it is part of a wider policy strategy, of isolating imprisoned populations from any communication with the outside world. In the recent typhoon in Burma, for example, the military government prevented American relief supplies from being delivered to populations in rural, difficult-to-access areas. This form of xenophobia and national isolation is reminiscent of the tactics the Communists used under Stalin, towards both their own citizens and "victim states" behind the "Iron Curtain." In the case of Burma, however, the government chose to sacrifice its own civilians rather than allow any form of exposure to the "free world."

Another example of state-controlled activity that resulted in untold suffering occurred after the Chernobyl nuclear power plant disaster. It exposed hundreds of thousands of civilians in the Ukraine to lethal doses of radiation—a catastrophe that largely could have been averted if the authorities had communicated with the citizens and implemented rescue protocols. Other examples of this kind of tragic situation abound. In the Sudan and Somalia, hundreds of thousands of civilians have starved to death while relief supplies have rotted because tribal warlords blocked access to them as part of their programs of ethnic genocide. In North Korea, starvation also remains rampant because the nation has been placed into forced isolation by the design of a mad dictator. In Zimbabwe, the entire nation stands on the brink of starvation due to a single man's obsession, President Robert Mugabe, to "nationalize" all farms. The lucrative, private, agricultural enterprises exported produce to the entire African continent and provided safe homesteads for thousands of black workers. Within a few years after the forceful removal of white landowners, the "bread-basket" of Africa was transformed into a wasteland. I know this first-hand from my father, who was born and grew up in Rhodesia.

Other examples of activities associated with state-terrorism include the rigging of elections, intimidation of voters, and attacks on civilians who advocate peaceful reform. Relief or rescue operations designed to disrupt such abuses of power and privilege are effective only if they address the root causes of the problems. At times, reform requires regime change, such as the ousting of Saddam Hussein in Iraq by the "Coalition of the Willing."

Once resources are in place, societies can approach the resumption of natural growth and seek strategies for social, psychological, and social healing. To gain access to resources, however, abusive governments have to be convinced that democratic governments will collectively unite to confront tyranny wherever it occurs.

The Reemergence of Soviet Imperialism

The recent Russian conquest of Georgia left the West appearing quite perplexed and ineffectual. The Russians borrowed their methodology from old KGB constructs of controlling victims using overwhelming power—a method used during the old days of the Cold War to subdue Czechoslovakia, Hungary and other Eastern European countries. In that process, the Soviets made every attempt to strip those countries of their national identities and have them submit to a "Central Power."

If ever there was a "State of Terror" it existed behind the "Iron Curtain." Since the intellectual mainstream exposed the propaganda template of Marxism as rubbish, they needed to fabricate a new one: Ossetia.

Propaganda attempts to conceal the real agenda of tyranny. The *continuous threat paradigm* is a useful model to explain the motive behind Russia's recent invasion of Georgia. Predators always try to isolate their victims, thereby removing their access to external resources and assistance. The victims' single most important behavior to stave-off severe anxiety and panic is the ability to communicate with significant others. Why did the Soviets need to dissect Georgia in half and destroy their communication systems? Was it not to achieve the goal of isolation?

I raise this point because it highlights the function of *caretaking* to a global level. Showing empathy towards a predator represents the first breakage of caretaking failure. Is there any correlation between "collective caretaking" failure and the Russian invasion of Georgia? If so, we may not have long to bask in the comfort of the post-Cold War Era.

Fear has a cross-sensitizing effect, so if Russia's other neighbors want to get too democratic or "cozy" with the West, then they might have to pay a price. The U.N. has thus far not even presented a motion condemning Russia's invasion of a neighboring sovereign state.

If there is anything to learn from history, Western Europe still has to define whether it has the will and means to protect itself. If not, as its recent antics suggest, then the world is heading toward being a much more dangerous place.

The War Against Jihad

Honest debate and the marketplace of public dialogue are antithetical to the methodology of Jihad. While we naively negotiate in good faith, based on a code of values, radical Islam sees the opportunity to negotiate through an entirely different prism. Indeed, they have mastered the skill of exploiting the vast network of mass media to constellate and even attract a wide appeal for genocide.

In the case of Jihad, terrorism was first given legitimacy and palatability by the real predator presenting himself as the victim. Fabricated scenes of wounded children, for example, drowned out the reality that missiles were deliberately fired from schools into populated civilian areas. At the same time hundreds of children were recruited for their army of suicide "martyrs."

While the true victims' mothers mourn, suicide-bombers' mothers celebrate. This propaganda hoax has generally been quite successful, especially to the European audience. The main achievement of this ploy has been its appeal to the mainstream media to promote and advertise the predator's "grievances." By not recognizing the success of the terrorists in gaining mass sympathy for total fabrications, Western nations—which pride themselves on truth and integrity—have virtually been taken intellectual hostage by the misguided lies that underpin the terrorists' ideology of hatred and intolerance.

Even elite centers of learning use "cross-cultural debates" as a front for pedantic hate-filled demagoguery. The effect has been a collective affliction of the "Stockholm Syndrome," whereby both victims and the world-wide audience become so identified with the "plight" of *predators* that they shed their own belief systems. In its place, empirical historical truths become replaced by the ideologies blindly imposed on them by predators, which become hijacked by those of the predators. The popular media have in fact, led the charge by the "extreme left" in garnishing support for radical Islam. In my opinion, this has been so effective because it constellates the latent anti-Semitism of the collective unconscious. The culmination of this process will be the ultimate success of political terrorism.

Aside from participation in this "propaganda delusion" by European audiences, Islamic terrorists have found another unexpected ally: the Government of Israel. As a result of caretaker failure, Israel's recent (experimental) "Government of Conciliation" sacrificed a major foreign policy priority to maintain neutral neighbors as protective buffer states. Judea, Sumaria, the Sinai, and Lebanon were always regarded by the Israeli defense establishment as providing vital strategic depth. During the Yom Kippur War, it was that strategic depth that saved it from total eradication.

Within months of shifting its policy to one of appeasement, its porous borders have become a national security nightmare.

Using the caretaker analogy, Iran and its terrorist proxies function as the "predator," Russia, China, Korea, and Pakistan as the "sponsors," while Western Europe plays its usual role as the colluding "caretaker." The United Nations, instead of functioning as a neutral power broker, has become the age-old *enabler*, providing the "town hall" as a podium for the promotion of its favored clients.

The net effect of this silent conspiracy has been the affliction of immense misery on both Jews and Arabs in the Middle East.

Jungian Archetypes and Political Terrorism

Islamic fascism, one of today's global predatorial forces, has a far-reaching infrastructure that disseminates its ideology through a multitude of Western media outlets. This predatorial stereotype is identified by Carl Jung as an archetype that he termed "The Trickster." It is discussed in detail by Edward Edinger, one of the founding members of the C.G. Jung Foundation, in his classic book *Ego and Archetype*.

Western democracies, on a peaceful footing following centuries of war, prefer to turn a blind eye to fascism and its contempt toward democratic values. As a result, according to John Bolton, former U.S. Ambassador to the U.N., Europe is effectively colluding with predators. Most Western media-outlets are attracted to the compelling propaganda template of a predator who stages himself as the *victim*.

This "role-reversal" is an essential template of the archetypal "Trickster," and is even found in the writings of the Prophet Muhammad: "War is won by deception."

Western democracies cannot exert a "caretaking role" against an "enemy" they do not perceive as such. While the Western left-liberal mindset has placed "tolerance" as sacrosanct, the predator views this as weakness, not friendship.

Students of object relations and geo-politics, however, understand this capitulation by the West as a form of caretaker failure. The consequences have yet to be seen, but they do not bode well.

The political implication of this reality is that governments need to understand that Islam is on the march, and much thought has to be devoted to containing it. Their doctrine of religious hatred and intolerance has to be abolished and replaced with models of critical thinking and the willingness to self-reflect. Journalism also has to re-invent itself, guided by models of truth, objectivity, and integrity. Watchdog groups have to hold the media responsible for upholding standards of integrity. Distortions in the reporting of events and journalistic bias need to become more transparent and responsible.

Government Accountability

Rapid rescue interventions have to be made available to the victims of political tyranny. Recent examples of civilian trauma candidates for such assistance include the crises in Burma and Georgia, where the obstruction of external rescue constituted an important component in the abuse against helpless civilians.

The compounding effects of prolonged social disruption, loss of family or community, constant danger, and unavailability of physical necessities constitute the *"continuous trauma paradigm"* (a term coined by Arieh Shalev in the article "Psychological Responses to Continuous Terror: A Study of Two Communities in Israel," published in the *American Journal of Psychiatry*). I mention this to indicate the breakdown of the caretaking function by a government under siege that was elected by a voting populace worn down by fear.

Elected governmental caretakers have to work collaboratively to protect their vital institutions against any attack on their culture or religion by establishing doctrines of self-preservation. All societies need to establish a mechanism that can rapidly remove any government that betrays these values. Democratic process is sacred, but not more so than life itself.

In the article I previously quoted by Savjak, regarding the Balkan Wars, the risk of PTSD resulting from the compounding effects of civil chaos in the face of international apathy approximated 42 percent.

Irwin Cotler, a professor of human rights and constitutional law at McGill University, has addressed the failure of caretaking at an international level in an article published in the August 1, 2008 issue of the *Jerusalem Post*. He describes the current crises as "the crime of indifference and inaction," and notes that, in spite of a lot of rhetoric on Darfur, 450,000 people have already died. He adds, "The killing fields have not abated." Our generation has witnessed ethnic cleansing in the Balkans, genocide in Rwanda, and the incitement to genocide by President Ahmadinejad of Iran.

It is important to emphasize here that while Iran and China have enjoyed immunity from condemnation in the United Nations, all 10 resolutions passed by the UN Human Rights Council in its first year of inception were against Israel.

It is ultimately the responsibility of the UN Security Council, the International Atomic Energy Agency (IAEA), and the International Criminal Court to honestly fulfill their role to prevent the escalation of terrorism, the nuclear pursuits of rogue states, human rights violations, and ethnic purging.

In this context, John Bolton noted that the prevailing dangers facing the U.S. included the internal strife within the Bush Administration, the policy of appeasement toward Europe, and the dissolution of the "Transatlantic Alliance." In his 2007 *New York Times* best-seller *Surrender Is Not an Option*, Bolton exposed in meticulous detail how U.S. negotiators were constantly betrayed by "behind-closed-doors" cloak-and-dagger obstructionism and foot-dragging orchestrated by Germany, France, and even the U.K.

Ironically, in the interest of appeasing Iran, Russia, and China, both the former UN Secretary Kofi Annan and the International Atomic Energy Board Director el Baraidi demonstrated a selective apathy toward confronting favored rogue states such as Iran and Pakistan.

The international community has to rebuild a doctrine based on the higher moral cause of "collective caretaking." Using a trauma model, governmental agencies as well as international agencies are crucial for maintaining a safe holding environment that allows ordinary citizens to live free of threat. This political failure of rescue and caretaking functions continues to endanger the lives of millions.

Chapter 6

WHAT HAPPENS TO THE BRAIN IN PTSD?

The Hippocampus, Hypothalamus, and Pituitary Glands

Physiologically, the part of the brain that functions as the "fear center" is the Amygdala. In contrast, the Hippocampus functions as a switch and "control center."

In primates (including human beings), the Hippocampus is the most complex and *delicate* part of the brain. It is a relatively small, deeply embedded body of neurons, in close proximity to the *emotional circuits* (also known as the limbic structures) and the "*Master-Endocrine Glands*," known as the Hypothalamus and Pituitary.

These endocrine brain structures, sitting right below the emotional limbic areas, are called "Master Glands" because they release hormonal proteins and other neurotransmitters that flow downstream and activate hormonal glands and neural networks throughout the body.

The lateral hypothalamus activates over-arousal of the sympathetic nervous centers in both the brain stem and spinal cord. Via spinal outlets, the adrenal glands are stimulated to produce adrenaline—the hormone responsible for the psychological sense of dread —and various accompanying physiological symptoms such as sweating, tightness of the chest, gastro-intestinal symptoms, and a rapid heart beat.

The medial hypothalamus is responsible for the production of Glucocorticoid Releasing Factor, which travels a short distance to the pituitary gland. There it stimulates the production of ACTH (adrenocorticoid-trophic hormone), which enters the bloodstream and activates the adrenal gland to produce cortisol.

This Hypothalamic-Pituitary-Adrenal axis activation is the biological signature of all stress. In PTSD, however, the system remains "turned on" well after the immediate stress has subsided, and specific trauma triggers easily reactivate it.

One sees from this process that both adrenaline and cortisol are involved in mediating stress responses.

The Hippocampus and Memory

The function of the Hippocampus is to link events to memory, tag them to an emotion, and then file these memorized events into an emotional narrative in the Temporal Lobe of the brain. Later, the Hippocampus is called upon to retrieve these recollections when faced with a similar threat. For adaptive purposes, memories associated with strong emotional content are more strongly consolidated and more easily accessed.

The release of large amounts of cortisol from the adrenal glands returns to the Hippocampus. Initially, it facilitates the Hippocampus to "over-memorize" traumatic events. But if the cortisol (together with other transmitters, such as glutamate) over-production continues, it causes the Hippocampal cells to degenerate and eventually die (apoptosis).

Detrimental Effects of Cortisol

Studies have shown that when rodents have their adrenal glands removed and are then subjected to stress their Hippocampus remains normal. This means that the presence of cortisol at the Hippocampal receptor is critical to the cascade leading to neuronal cell death. This explains that the complexity of the Hippocampus is commensurate with its sensitivity to the toxic effects of stress-generated hormones, including cortisol and glutamic acid.

The Hippocampus plays a role in providing memory with context and emotional relevance. It also restrains the Amygdala from activating fear responses while notifying the prefrontal brain of response-choices that are far more diverse and receptive to modification, when comparing humans with other primates.

Protective Mechanisms and Negative Feedback Loops

The understanding that trauma activates the Hypothalamic-Pituitary-Adrenal Axis has been confounded by the unexpected low levels of cortisol in the body fluids of traumatized populations. This apparent contradiction is explained as follows: The Amygdala, which is the center of your *fear circuitry,* will continue to produce large amounts of CRF if you have PTSD. The Pituitary gland had to "protect itself" by dynamically changing certain neuronal receptors to apply a "brake system." Brake systems express themselves in the brain by way of receptors delivering a message to the DNA of the cell. In this case, if you have PTSD, the traumatic injury has activated a sustained *fear response.* The DNA in the Hypothalamus, as a protective device, is informed by its glucocortisoid receptor to produce fewer CRF receptors.

This is one way the brain attempts to switch down cortisol production. CRF is the first step in the chain of hormonal stress responses.

Several studies have, indeed, shown that stressed individuals downregulate their pituitary CRF receptors. They therefore respond sluggishly in their production of ACTH when stimulated by CRF. The downstream effect is to discourage the adrenal glands from releasing cortisol.

The second mechanism has to do with your pituitary gland and its "negative-feedback" mechanism mediated by cortisol autoreceptors. Since your body "knows" that prolonged exposure to high cortisol is "bad," your cortisol (glucocortisoid) receptors become "upregulated." This is because these receptors function as a "negative feedback loop" to "switch down" the production of ACTH from an over-stimulated pituitary. The Glucocorticoid receptor functions as a messenger, warning the cell to prevent more production of ACTH. Your body is trying to prevent the inevitable cascade that would lead to the second step in the production of cortisol.

If you have PTSD, your pituitary gland is receiving two conflicting messages: CRF from the Amygdala and Hypothalamus is demanding the production of ACTH, but the upregulated Glucocortisoid receptor tries to prevent this from happening, via a negative feedback loop to reduce the production of ACTH.

The usual winner in this "tug-of-war" is the negative counter-responses. The net result of this tug-of-war may even lead to a *decreased* production of ACTH and cortisol. This finding initially caught the scientific world by surprise, because some stressed and traumatized individuals were showing *lower levels of cortisol* in their blood and saliva. Some investigators quickly went to test this negative feedback hypothesis.

Testing the Negative Feedback Loop Hypothesis

Metyrapone is a substance that *blocks* cortisol synthesis. Administering metyrapone will, therefore, eliminate any negative-feedback effect of cortisol on the Pituitary Gland. In one study, victims of combat and rape who were given metyrapone *showed much more elevation* of ACTH and cortisol than control subjects (Yehuda, 1996). In other words, once the negative feedback loop of cortisol has been removed, CRF becomes free to stimulate the Pituitary, unimpeded by cortisol's opposing (negative feedback) effect at the upregulated Glucocorticoid receptor site. This study was replicated sufficiently to convince investigators that *cortisol levels per se* are a *poor marker* for the diagnosis of PTSD.

Another test works in the opposite direction: Stressed victims show blunted responses of ACTH when given dexamethasone, a potent Glucocorticoid. In other words, if you have PTSD, you will produce less ACTH when given a potent Glucocortisoid, because of upregulation of your cortisol-mediated brakes applied to your ACTH-producing cells. Naive control subjects don't have upregulated negative feedback loop receptors. So when healthy volunteers receive dexamethasone, there is a measured suppression by the pituitary of ACTH. But once trauma has upregulated the protective negative feedback loops, dexamethasone has an exaggerated suppression on cortisol production (see Goenjian, 1995).

At first the findings of lower-than-expected cortisol in abuse victims was extremely counter-intuitive. We first had to understand that there is a protective mechanism guarding the Hypothalamic-Pituitary-Adrenal axis. The body appears to "know" how dangerous cortisol can be to the Hippocampus.

As long as PTSD remains untreated, a problem remains, in that the Hypothalamic-Pituitary-Adrenal axis is being simultaneously stimulated (by increased CRF) and restrained (by hypersensitivity to normal or even low cortisol in the blood). In an automobile, this would be like pushing the gas pedal and the brakes at the same time!

The continued state of this dynamic conflict has an obvious "wear-and-tear" effect on the entire above-mentioned neuroendocrine system if PTSD is not treated. This expresses itself in the body via somatic and other stress-related symptoms, including fatigue and increased stress on the immune and cardiovascular systems.

The Role of Hippocampal Failure in the Pathogenesis of PTSD

It is not difficult to conclude that, when the Hippocampus is *overwhelmed* by stress-induced neurotoxins such as glutamate, glucocortisoid, or its precursor, Glucocortisoid Releasing Factor (GRF), it shuts down. In fact, Functional MRI studies have demonstrated immediate Hippocampal impairment in the immediate aftermath of rape (see Debellis et al., 2000).

What then occurs is a cascading sequence of events where frightening sensory images are left free-floating. In the absence of a viable Hippocampal "librarian" function, raw fragments of trauma imagery, unable to be "filed" in an orderly way, continue the downward neuroendocrine cascade of continued trauma activation. This phenomenon is sometimes refereed to as "kindling" or "sensitization."

The resulting effect of the dual *over-activation* of the Amygdala and *paralysis* of the Hippocampus provides the neurobiological substrate for most of the observed symptoms in PTSD.

The Trauma Cascade

Traumatizing experiences have a tendency to generalize and sensitize the trauma survivor to a wide array of threat cues. Trauma violates safety assumptions. Situations previously considered safe become danger signals. This increases the likelihood that you will be constantly scanning the world around you to identify threat. Your *Sympathetic Nervous System* is constantly on the alert. In this state of activated threat arousal, there is a greater likelihood of interpreting ambiguous information as dangerous.

While identifying and treating PTSD has always been the priority in treating survivors of abuse, only recently have modalities been developed that target the deleterious effects of continued overarousal. In such a state of activated threat arousal, it is impossible to process traumatic memories in a constructive or therapeutic way. From a psychological perspective, if you are unable to self-soothe and lack the skill to be sufficiently "anchored and mindful," then synthesizing a coherent trauma-narrative becomes all the more difficult.

At a biological level, when the activated Amygdala is producing excessive amounts of CRF, this combines with other toxic neurotransmitters, such as cortisol and glutamate, causing the Hippocampus to shut down. As previously mentioned, this is the key brain structure required to assist the victim to re-visit the trauma and appropriately contextualize it. Medications that have a calming effect, as well as behavioral calming techniques, have been shown to restore Hippocampal viability in traumatized individuals and animals.

GLOSSARY

Acute Stress Disorder: A disruption in the integrated flow of consciousness of some survivors within hours or days after they have a shocking experience. They often have significant dissociation and difficulty in their day-to-day functioning because of uncontrolled arousal as well as flashbacks. This condition may be the early precursor of PTSD.

Amnesia: One of the symptoms of dissociation whereby a traumatized victim has difficulty recalling the traumatic event.

Amygdala: A series of nuclear masses located on the medial portion of the temporal lobe of the brain. It fuses with the caudate and putamen (involved with motor tone and motility) on the medial side and the Hippocampus on the lateral side. Lesions in the Amygdala of animals have a "taming effect." Stimulation, however, results in heightened startle responses, increased blood pressure and heart rate, and production of acid in the stomach, which can cause ulcers. It is, therefore, regarded as the epicenter of fear-mediated responses.

Avoidance: One of the cardinal symptoms of PTSD. Avoidance refers either to ego defenses or inhibiting behaviors that shelter an individual against distressing thoughts, memories, or emotions. "Instrumental learning" involves engaging in behaviors that improve well-being by escaping from painful memories and fear-triggers. While in some circumstances this leads to adaptive survival, it can also interfere with a wide range of stress exposure required for social and occupational functioning.

Caretaker: A person or agency responsible for the care of another human being, especially during infancy and early socialization. When this term is applied to the syndrome of abuse, "caretaker failure" is a serious contributing factor. Adequate caretaking involves an asymmetric but caring relationship between someone more powerful and another who is more vulnerable. In childhood, parents usually provide emotional and physical safe-haven. In societies, agencies provide supportive services for individuals at risk, such as for the elderly and infirm. At a governmental level a "defense force" is charged with the responsibility of defending citizens against foreign attack.

Cognitive Behavior Theory: Several studies have corroborated the efficacy of cognitive techniques in treating PTSD and Complex Trauma. These include "anchoring" and "mindfulness." This method advanced far beyond simple "exposure" that allows the individual to habituate to repeated trauma narration. It allows the victim to identify all trauma triggers, their effect on his or her thoughts, affects, and behaviors, and provides strategies to replace them with more adaptive ones.

Complex Trauma: Following Julian Ford, this syndrome is a unique response to prolonged, interpersonal captivity that is distinct from but overlaps with PTSD. First described by Judith Herman, it affects core personality factors and produces symptoms such as a deformed sense of perception and meaning, guilt, shame, chronic pain, dysfunctional mood regulation, and re-victimization in future relationships. Unlike pure PTSD, therefore, Complex Trauma affects core functions of personality structure without requiring the fear, vigilance, and avoidance behaviors that characterize PTSD. Complex Trauma is also referred to as "Disorder of Extreme Stress Not Otherwise Specified" (DESNOS).

CRF (Corticotrophin Releasing Factor): Investigators believe CRF is the crucial link between life-stress and the development of subsequent psychopathology. It has been found to be elevated in the cerebrospinal fluid of patients suffering from PTSD, as well as in animals exposed to adverse early rearing.

Dialectic Behavior Therapy: A treatment philosophy originally developed by Dr. Marsha Linehan for treating patients with "Borderline Personality Disorder." It now dominates the rationale for the cognitive behavioral management of trauma survivors. It is heavily influenced by the Zen school of Eastern spiritual training, but is compatible with Western contemplation and meditation practices. It replaces the "emotional mind," where thoughts or behaviors are distorted by fear or anger, with the "wise mind," which is focused and present.

Disorder of Extreme Stress Not Otherwise Specified (DESNOS). See Complex Trauma.

Dissociation: A common reaction to severe trauma. It ranges from being confused and disoriented, in its acute form, to being emotionally detached or even "absent," in survivors of prolonged interpersonal trauma.

Dissociative Identity Disorder: A serious, traumatically induced split of the personality into different identities (formerly termed "Multiple Personality Disorder").

Emotional Regulation: One's capacity to tolerate all kinds of emotional feelings without resorting to outbursts of anger, excessive avoidance, or over-reliance on substances. Strategies for learning how to handle unpleasant emotions are acquired in early relationships with empathic caretakers (usually parents).

Flashback: A sudden, vivid recollection of any past trauma. It can occur spontaneously or following exposure to some reminder of the trauma.

Fugue State. A severe form of dissociation in which survivors, following horrific events, are unable to identify themselves.

Glucocortioids: Steroids released by the adrenal glands during stress. They exert a toxic effect and even cell death, however, which account in part for the findings of decreased Hippocampal volume in patients with PTSD.

Glutamate: The most important of the "Excitatory Amino Acids." In chronic stress, high cortisol levels, in conjunction with rapid glutamate "volleys," contribute to cell injury and death observed in the Hippocampus.

Hippocampus: A limbic structure located on the medial wall of the temporal lobe of the brain. The Hippocampal formation takes part in multiple activities, including endocrine production, learning, memorizing, expression of emotion, and autonomic functions such as establishing sympathetic or parasympathetic dominance. Because of an inborn, protective, negative feedback loop and receptor regulation, prednisone injections have an inhibiting effect on neurons in the Hippocampus. It has recently been established that the Hippocampus constrains the Amygdala from activating fear responses.

Pituitary: Referred to as the "master Endocrine Gland," because its hormones flow downstream to activate the entire endocrine system. Such hormones include Growth Hormone, prolactin, Thyroid-Stimulating Hormone (TSH), Follicular-Stimulating-Hormone (FSH), and Adrenocorticoid Hormone (ACTH).

Post-traumatic Stress Disorder (PTSD): Now considered as one of the cardinal (but not the exclusive) categories of stress-induced pathology. Following confrontation with a life-threatening event, if a victim feels horrified and has persistent stress symptoms, he or she may have developed full-blown PTSD. The neurobiology of this condition is explained in the text. The essential symptoms consist of reliving the trauma, over-vigilance, and avoidance behavior.

Psychodynamic Therapy: While Freud's theory of defenses is a useful construct that explains how the ego protects itself against painful trauma recollections, and is the purpose of avoidance, there is only scanty evidence that this form of therapy cures any of the trauma syndromes.

Schemas: Mental "models" based primarily on significant early relationships that shape our future relationships with others. In

Cognitive Therapy, recovery focuses on abuse schemas where the victim re-enacts his or her early abuse.

Self-Agency: Healthy self-regard and the ability both to creatively engage the present and stand up for one's rights. It often fails to develop in victims of chronic interpersonal abuse. Loss of self-agency is frequently found in victims of childhood abuse. Ongoing political terrorism can create an environment of fear and intimidation whereby victims cannot make choices that appear to be free, whether social, political, or religious.

Self-Object: The infant's internalized experience of the primary caretaker (usually the parent), which becomes part of the infant's sense of itself. Before the infant has established its own sense of self, it depends on a healthy supply of external emotional validation and empathic responses from the primary caretaker. This is what Franz Kohut calls the "good self-object."

Self-Psychology: The therapeutic process by which the therapist pays close attention to the client's inner state. Unlike classic psychoanalysis, this therapy requires an effort from the therapist to "get in touch" empathically with the client's inner experience. From a "transference" perspective, this process mirrors the validation of early good "self-object" experiences. When this method is employed with trauma survivors, they feel soothed, more cohesive, and less frightened and vulnerable than they are apt to feel with other therapeutic methods.

Self-Soothing: Early bonding and empathic attachments that shape one's sense of safety and well being throughout life. Children internalize the mood states of parents, which maintain their sense of well being during later stress. If a child experienced adequate soothing in early life and was not abused, then he or she can rekindle those good "self-objects" later in life.

Sympathetic Nervous System: That part of the nervous system that becomes activated by stress. In traumatized victims, the activation can help mobilize rescue-responses. When activation is excessive or prolonged, it explains much of the underlying neurobiological mechanisms in patients with post-traumatic stress disorder (PTSD).

Type I Trauma: This trauma results from a single, catastrophic event. Depending on the resilience of the victim and the severity of the trauma, the individual may experience an array of symptoms, ranging from worry and apprehension to PTSD.

Type II Trauma: This trauma is usually of a prolonged or recurrent and interpersonal type. Examples include victims of domestic violence or battered victims. Rather than causing acute stress, symptoms involve long-lasting alterations in emotional regulation, distortions in meaning and perceptions, and alterations in relationships with others.

REFERENCES

Bleich, A., Gelkopf, M., & Solomon, Z. (2003). Exposure to terrorism, stress-related mental health symptoms, and coping behaviors among a nationally representative sample in Israel. *JAMA, 290,* 612-620.

Bolton, John. (2007). *Surrender is not an option. Defending America at the United Nations and Abroad.* New York: Simon and Schuster/Threshold Editions.

Bremner, J. (1999). Alterations in brain structure and function associated with post-traumatic stress disorder. *Semin Clin Neuropsychiatry 4*:249-55.

Bremner, J.D., Licinio, J., Darnell, A., Krystal, J.H., Owens, M.J., Southwick, S.M., (1997). Elevated CSF Corticotropin-Releasing Factor concentrations in posttraumatic stress disorder. *Am J Psychiatry 154*:624-9.

Bremner, J.D., Randall, P., Vermetten, E., Staib, L., (1997). Magnetic resonance imaging-based measurement of Hippocampal volume in posttraumatic stress disorder related to childhood physical and sexual abuse—A preliminary report. *Biol Psychiatry 41*:23-32

Brewin, C. (2005). Systematic review of screening instruments for adults at risk of post traumatic stress disorder. *Journal of Traumatic Stress, 18*(1): 53-62.

Cheung P. (1994). Posttraumatic stress disorder among Cambodian refugees in New Zealand. *Int. J Soc Psychiatry 40*(1): 17-26.

Cloitre, M., Cohen, L.R., & Koenen, C.K. (2006). *Treating survivors of childhood abuse: Psychotherapy for the interrupted life*. New York: The Guilford Press.

Cloitre, M., Koenen, K., Cohen, L,.R., & Han, H. (2001). Skills training in affective and interpersonal regulation followed by exposure: A phase-based treatment for PTSD related to childhood abuse. *Journal of Consulting and Clinical Psychology, 70*(5), 1067-1074.

Cotler, Irwin. (2008, August 1-7). Global legal mind. *The International Jerusalem Post.*

Cohen-Silver, R., Holman, A., McIntosh, D.N., Poulin, M., Gil-Rivas, V., (2002). Nationwide longitudinal study of psychological responses to September 11. *JAMA, 288*: 1235-1244.

Curran, P.S. (1988). Psychiatric aspects of terrorist violence: Northern Ireland 1969-1987. *British J Psychiatry 153: 470-475.*

Davis, M. (1997). Neurobiology of fear responses: The role of the amygdala. *J. Neuropsychiatry Clin. Neurosci., 9*: 382-402.

De Bellis, M.D., Keshavan, M.S., Spencer, S., & Hall, J. (2000). N-Acetylaspartate concentration in the anterior cingulate of maltreated children and adolescents with PTSD. *Am J Psychiatry 157*(7): 1175-7.

De Kloet, E. R., Azmitia, E. C., & Landfield, P. W. (Eds.). (1996). Brain corticosteroid receptors: Studies on the mechanism, function, and neurotoxicity of corticosteroid action. *Ann. N.Y. Acad. Sci., 746*:1-499.

Diagnostic and statistical manual of mental disorders, 4th ed. (DSM-IV). (1994). Washington, DC: American Psychiatric Press.

Edinger, E. (1992). *Ego and archetype*. NY: Shambhala Press.

Elson, Miriam (Ed.). (1987). *The Kohut seminars on self psychology and psychotherapy with adolescents and young adults.* New York: W.W. Norton.

Foa, E. B., Keane, T. M., & Friedman, M. J. E. (Eds.). (2000). *Effective treatments for PTSD. Practice guidelines from the International Society for Traumatic Stress Studies.* New York: Guilford Press.

Foa, E. B., Riggs, D. S., Massie, E. D. & Yarczower, M., (1995). The impact of fear activation and anger on the efficacy of exposure treatment for posttraumatic stress disorder. *Behavior Therapy, 26,* 487-499.

Freyd, J. J. (1996). *Betrayal trauma, the logic of forgetting childhood abuse.* Cambridge, MA: Harvard University Press.

Ford, Julian. (1999). Disorders of extreme stress following war-zone military trauma: Associated features of PTSD or comorbid but distinct syndromes. *Journal of Consulting* & Clinical Psychology, 67(1): 3-12.

Ford, Julian & Kidd, Phyllis. (1998). Early childhood trauma and disorders of extreme stress as predictors of treatment outcome with chronic posttraumatic stress disorder. *Journal of Traumatic Stress, 11*(4): 743-761.

Greenacre, P. (1958). Early physical determinants in the development of the sense of identity. *Journal of the American Psychoanalytic Association, 6*: 612-27.

Greenberg, J. R, & Mitchell, S. A. (1983). *Object relations in psychoanalytic theory.* Cambridge, MA: Harvard University Press.

Herman, Judith. (1999). *Trauma and recovery: The aftermath of violence—from domestic violence to political terror.* New York: Basic Books.

Herman, Judith. (1992). Complex PTSD: A syndrome in survivors of prolonged and repeated trauma. *Journal of Traumatic Stress, 5*, 377-392.

Jacobson, L. & Sapolsky, R. (1991). The role of the hippocampus in feedback regulation of the hypothalamic-pituitary adrenocortical axis. *Endocrinol. Rev. 12*:118-134.

Jones, J. & Barlow, D. (1990). The etiology of post-traumatic stress disorder. *Clinical Psychological Review, 10:* 299-328.

Kernberg, Otto. (1998). Pathological narcissism and narcissistic personality disorder. In Elsa F. Ronningstam (ed.), *Disorders of narcissism* (pp. 37-41).

Kinzie, J.D., Boehnlein, J. K., Riley, C., & Sparr, L. (2002). The effects of September 11 on traumatized refugees: Reactivation of posttraumatic stress disorder. *J Nerv Ment Dis., 190*(7): 437-41.

Kohut, H. (1977). *The Restoration of the self. Does psychoanalysis need a psychology of the self?* New York: International Universities Press Inc.

LeDoux, J. E., Iwata, J., Cicchetti-V., & Reis, D. J. (1998). Different projections of the central amygdaloid nucleus mediate autonomic and behavioral correlates of conditioned fear. *J. of Neurosci. 8*: 2517-2529.

Linehan, M. M. (1993). *Skills training manual for treating borderline personality disorder.* New York: The Guilford Press.

McNally, R. J., Kaspi, S. P., Riemann, B. C., Zeitlin, S. B. (1990). Selective processing of threat cues in posttraumatic stress disorder. *J Abnorm Psychol, 99*:398-402.

Mahler, M. (1974). Symbiosis and individuation: The psychological birth of the human infant. In the *Selected papers of Margaret S. Mahler, Volume 2*. New York: Jason Erinson.

Mahler, M. (1971). Study of the separation individuation process and its possible application to borderline phenomena in the psychoanalytic situation. *Psychoanalytic Study of the Child, 26.*

Masterson, J. & Klein, R. (1995). *Disorders of the self: The Masterson approach.* New York: Brunner/Mazel, Inc.

Mollica, R.F., McKinnes, K., Sarajic, N. (1998). *Trauma and disability: Long term recovery of Bosnian refugees.* Cambridge: Harvard Program in Refugee Trauma.

Pelcovitz, D., Van Der Kolk, M., Roth, S., Mandel, F., Kaplan, S., Resick, P., (1997). Development of a criteria set and a structured interview for disorders of extreme stress (SIDES). *Journal of Traumatic Stress,10*(1): 3-16.

Phillips, R. G. & LeDoux, J. E. (1992). Differential contribution of amygdala and hippocampus to cued and contextual fear conditioning. *Behav. Neurosci., 106*:247-285.

Roozdaal, B., Nguyen, B., Power, A., & McGaugh, J. (1999). Basolateral amygdala noradrenergic influence enables enhancement of memory consolidation by hippocampal glucocorticoid receptor activation. *Proc Natl Sci USA, 96*(11): 642-47.

Rubin, G. J., Brewin, C. R., Greenberg, N., Simpson, J., Wessely, S., (2005). Psychological and behavioral reactions to the bombings in London on 7 July 2005: Cross sectional survey of a representative sample of Londoners. *British Medical Journal, 331:* 606-612.

Savjak, N. (2003). Multiple traumatisation as a risk factor of post-traumatic stress disorder. *PSIHOLOGIJA, 36*(1-2): 59-71.

Schlenger, W. E., Caddell, J. M., Ebert, L., Jordan, B.K., Rourke, K.M., Wilson, D. (2002). Psychological reactions to terrorist attacks: Findings from the national study of Americans' reactions to September 11. *JAMA, 288*: 581-588.

Schuff, N., Marmar, C. R., Weiss, D. S., Neylan, T. C., Schoenfeld, F., Fein, G., & Weiner, M. W. (1997). Reduced hippocampal volume and n-acetyl aspartate in posttraumatic stress disorder. *Ann NY Acad Sci, 821*:516-20.

Schuster, M. A., Stein, B. D., Jaycox, L., Collins, R.L., Marshall, G.N., Elliott, M.N. (2001). A national survey of stress reactions after the September 11, 2001, terrorist attacks. *New Engl J Med, 345*:1507-1512.

Shalev, A., Tuval, R. A., Frenkiel-Fishman, S., Hadar, H., & Spencer, E. (2006). Psychological responses to continuous terror: A study of two communities in Israel. *American Journal of Psychiatry, 164*(4), 667-673.

Siegel, G. J. & Hartzell, M. (2003). *Parenting from the inside out. How a deeper self-understanding can help you raise children who thrive.* New York: Tarcher/Putnam.

Solomon, Z. & Prager, E. (1992). Elderly Israeli Holocaust survivors during the Persian Gulf War. *American Journal of Psychiatry, 149*(12), 1707-1710.

Stein, M. B., Koverola, C., Hanna, C., Torchia, M.G., McClarty, B., (1997). Hippocampal volume in women victimized by childhood sexual abuse. *Psychol Med, 27*:951-9.

Thich, Nhat Hanh. (1987). *The Miracle of mindfulness. An introduction to the practice of meditation.* Boston: Beacon Press.

Trappler, B. & Friedman, S. (1996). Post-traumatic stress in the survivors of the Brooklyn Bridge shooting. *American Journal of Psychiatry*, 153(5), 705-7.

Trappler, B. & Newville, H. (2007). Trauma healing via group cognitive behavior therapy in chronically hospitalized patients. *Psychiatric Quarterly, 78*(4):317-25.

U.S. Department of State: Bureau of Public Health (2005). Retrieved from the Internet December 2008 at https://www.state.gov/.

Vasquez, C., Perez-Sales, P., & Matt, G. (2006). Posttraumatic stress reactions following the March 11, 2004, terrorist attacks in a Madrid community sample. *The Spanish Journal of Psychology, 99*(1), 61-74.

Van Der Hart, O., Nijenhuis, E., & Steele, K. (2006). *The haunted self. Structural dissociation of chronic traumatization.* New York: W.W. Norton & Company.

Van Der Kolk, B. A. (1989). The compulsion to repeat trauma: Revictimization, attachment, and masochism. *The Psychiatric Clinics of North America, 12:* 389-411.

Van Der Kolk, B. A. & Fisler, R. (1995). Dissociation and the fragmentary nature of traumatic memories. *Journal of Traumatic Stress, 8:* 505-525.

Van Der Kolk, B. A., Pelcovitz, D., Roth, S., Mandel, F.S., McFarlane, A., & Herman, J. (1996). Dissociation, somatization, and affect dysregulation: The complexity of adaptation to trauma. *Am. J. Psychiatry, 153*(7): 83-93.

Van Der Kolk, B. A., Roth, S., Pelcovitz, D., Sunday, S., Spinazzola, J. (2005). Disorders of extreme stress: The empirical foundation of a complex adaptation to trauma. *Journal of Traumatic Stress*, 18(5).

Williams, M. B. & Poijula, S. (2002). *The PTSD workbook. Simple, effective techniques for overcoming traumatic stress symptoms.* Oakland, CA: New Harbinger Publications, Inc.

Winnicott, D. W. (1965). *The maturational process and the facilitating environment.* New York: International University Press.

Yehuda, R., Boisoneau, D., Lowy, M. T., & Giller, E.L. (1995). Dose-response changes in plasma cortisol and lymphocyte glucocorticoid receptors following dexamethasone administration in combat veterans with and without PTSD. *Arch Gen Psychiatry, 52*:583-93.

Yehuda, R., Kahana, B., Binder-Brynes, K., Southwick, S.M., Mason, J.W., & Giller, E.L. (1995). Low urinary cortisol excretion in Holocaust survivors with PTSD. *Am J Psychiatry, 152*: 982-6.

Yehuda, R., Levengood, R., Schmeidler, J., Wilson, S., Guo, L.S., & Gerber, D. (1996). Increased pituitary activation following metyrapone administration in PTSD. *Psychoneuroendocrinology, 21*:1-16.

Yehuda, R., Lowy, M. T., Southwick, S. M., Shaffer, D., & Giller, E.L. (1991). Lymphocyte glucocorticoid receptor number in PTSD. *Am J Psychiatry, 148*: 499-504.

INDEX